Pelican Books
The Pill on Trial

Paul Vaughan left Oxford in 1950 with a wartime
degree in French and an honours degree in English.
He quickly became involved with medicine and
doctors and worked for a time for a drug company
in Camberwell, exporting ointments and pep pills
to Africa and the near East. Subsequently he
joined the staff of the British Medical Association,
eventually becoming Chief Press Officer. In 1964
he left the BMA to devote himself to full-time
medical journalism. He also broadcasts regularly
on radio and television. In such time as there is
left he plays the clarinet and enjoys the countryside
in mid-Wales. He and his wife and four children have
a small farmhouse in Montgomeryshire and divide
their time unequally between that and their house in
Wimbledon.

PAUL VAUGHAN

# The Pill on Trial

PENGUIN BOOKS

Penguin Books Ltd, Harmondsworth,
Middlesex, England
Penguin Books Australia Ltd, Ringwood,
Victoria, Australia

First published by Weidenfeld & Nicolson 1970
Published in Pelican Books 1972

Made and printed in Great Britain by
C. Nicholls & Company Ltd
Set in Linotype Pilgrim

# Contents

# Preface to the Pelican Edition

By the end of 1971 the number of women in Britain using the pill had passed 1,800,000 and showed every sign of proceeding smoothly on beyond two million. Or, in other words, between 18 and 20 per cent of the women of child-bearing age in this country now prefer the pill to any other kind of contraceptive – a convincing demonstration, if such were needed, of the pill's attractiveness and convenience, not to mention its effectiveness.

One can also assume that nearly two million women have decided that the benefits and advantages of the pill count for more than its risks, in spite of the publicity given to the complicated and delicate question of safety, which might well have been a source of much greater discouragement. In fact, during the two years since this book first appeared, the side-effects of the pill have faded from public discussion. Faith in oral contraceptives has been quietly restored. Perhaps there is a residuum of anxiety capable of being stirred, but for the moment it is dormant, while the debate over the safety of the pill takes place, desultorily, in private.

Meanwhile research continues, much of it consisting of the steady amassing of information about the health of large numbers of women taking the pill over a period of years. In Britain the Royal College of General Practitioners is going on with its survey which follows the fortunes of 20,000 women, half of them users of the pill, half using other kinds of contraceptive. No warnings have been heard from doctors engaged in this and similar epidemiological studies, and one must assume that so far no evidence has emerged to justify a wholesale flight from the pill.

This is certainly true in the case of the dread possibility of a link between the pill and cancer, undoubtedly the most alarming of the side-effects being discussed while I was gathering material for *The Pill on Trial*. Nothing, in this respect, has been heard to amplify the suspicions referred to later in these pages. The link has not been substantiated and perhaps it never will be.

At the same time, the use of pills low on oestrogen appears to have reduced the number of fatal blood-clotting episodes among women on the pill. If there have been any sudden deaths from thromboembolism among pill-users they have remained unpublicized: coroners' comments on such tragic cases, for long a recurrent cause of failing confidence in the pill, are no longer to be read in the newspapers.

The 'mini-pill', too, is emerging from the cloud it was under during the bleak winter (for the pill and its makers) of 1969–70. Consisting of only one active drug (a progestogen) and not two, the mini-pill appeared to have numerous advantages over conventional contraceptive pills. Then, because of suspicious results from routine tests on beagle bitches, the mini-pill was hastily withdrawn by the drug firms manufacturing it. Too hastily, if some doctors are to be believed, but perhaps understandably so in the nervous atmosphere of that particular winter, when the Drug Safety Committee's advice that women should avoid high-oestrogen pills was widely misunderstood, and thought to be a warning of some new blood-clotting danger. And in due course the manufacturers themselves came round to the view that they had, perhaps, gone too far, and had read too much into the results of the animal experiments. New submissions went to the Drug Safety Committee. There now seems little reason why the mini-pill, in several varieties, should not be completely restored to favour.

So is the pill still on trial? There must remain a reasonable degree of scepticism about a drug so widely used day after day, and even in a culture that relies as heavily as ours on solace from the medicine bottle. The dose may be small in today's oral contraceptives, and it is indeed small compared with the powerful quantities swallowed by the obedient mothers of Puerto Rico in 1956. But magnitude is still comparative, and who can say whether even a dose measured in microgrammes would not have unlooked for consequences if consumed throughout most of a woman's child-bearing years? All one can say is that, for the moment, there is no evidence that any serious and irreversible ill effects are likely to follow. And even if there were, one would have to make some kind of personal assessment of how far they were outweighed by the attractiveness, convenience, and effectiveness of the pill – or at least make the attempt to do so.

My object in writing *The Pill on Trial* was not to supply a ready-made answer to this exceedingly difficult question. For the time being, as I have suggested here, there is no generally applicable answer, because we do not have all the facts at our disposal. What I have tried to do is to set out, for the record, the nature of the medical argument over the pill and its possible hazards – an argument that, as is the way in medicine, tends to spill over into questions of conscience, morality, and social justice. By the nature of things, the strictly medical aspects of the argument have not always been clearly understandable to the man in the street or, more appropriately, the woman in the supermarket. If the admirable doctrine of 'informed consent' hopefully pursued by Senator Gaylord Nelson (and described in the epilogue to this book) is to be brought within reach of the woman at risk, then there is an undeniable need for some such account as I have, I hope, been able to provide.

Wimbledon                                              P.V.
February 1972

# Acknowledgements

Much of the material for *The Pill on Trial* was collected in the course of conversations with men and women in Britain and the United States professionally concerned in one way or another with oral contraception – prescribers, research workers, committee men, manufacturers or advertisers. I have also had a great deal of help from the staffs of various official and semi-official bodies who willingly spared the time to talk about their work and to discuss the problems of the pill.

Some of the book was the result of talking to women who are, or have been, simply consumers, voices from the multitude of pill-takers, whose feelings on the subject often go unheard.

Without the help of all these people, this book could never have been written.

Grateful thanks are also due to those friends whose comments at various stages of the book have been invaluable: especially Stephen Lock, Derek Cooper, and Hilary Rubinstein, without whom the book would not have been started at all.

Special thanks must go to Susan Wijdenes, whose expert and diplomatic help in New York eliminated many of the obstacles in the way of an inexperienced visitor and also made geographical sense of an impossible visiting list.

To my brother David Vaughan special thanks must also go for his help in New York and for keeping me supplied with news of the pill which would otherwise have been hard to obtain.

But above all, thanks to my wife – fellow-traveller and fellow-sufferer, whose constant encouragement whether the book was going well or badly, has been beyond adequate acknowledgement.

# Introduction

Optimists can see in the story of the contraceptive pill one of the greatest boons ever conferred on humanity by science, a discovery which solves easily and agreeably the individual's problem of family spacing, and simultaneously offers a way of slowing down the frightening rate of population increase all over the world.

Pessimists see something else: a supreme example of scientific arrogance, with its reckless interference with a vital process of nature for the sake of a short-term gain, and its assumption that a mechanism as fundamental as human reproduction can be continuously put out of action by synthetic chemicals.

Between the two points of view are the women, nearly twenty million of them, who take the pill.

While collecting material for this book I have been reminded by people I have talked to of the responsibilities of journalists who write about the subject for public consumption. Doctors especially like to warn laymen off something they regard as too complicated, with too many traps for the uninformed and involving too many medical details which will needlessly alarm the pill-users. There is some truth in this, but any attempt to confine discussion of the pill to medical circles is doomed from the start. Like abortion, euthanasia, transplant surgery or the manipulation of genes, pill contraception demands public discussion.

I began work on this book with few preconceived ideas or, as far as I know, prejudices about the pill. I have no religious or conscientious scruples about the pill or any other method of contraception. I am not against sexual freedom either, and it seems necessary to say so if only because advocates of the pill sometimes imply that anyone who criticizes it must be against sex, an accusation usually good for a round of applause in public discussions.

One puzzling aspect of the subject, to me, is that so many

people have apparently found it easy to make up their minds whether the pill is a good thing or not. My sympathies are with the doctor who complained about the 'excessive polarization' of opinion. There are good things about the pill, and bad ones, and sooner or later society must make up its mind, with medical advice, which are the more important.

On all types of contraceptive pill now available there is a huge library of studies of the effectiveness, safety, side-effects, extent of use and comparative advantages of one pill over another. So voluminous is the literature that a complete bibliography of references has now ceased to be practicable. Although it has only been in existence for just over a dozen years, the contraceptive pill has been studied more extensively than any other drug in history. This can be used as an argument for the pill, or against it. It can be said that if we knew as much about aspirin and its side-effects as we know about oral contraceptives, we should have every right to be as apprehensive about its long-term effects. But, unlike aspirin, the pill is designed for continuous, chronic use, and the protean nature of its effects brought to light by this astonishing amount of investigation, calls for a different standard of safety.

The galloping increase in the world's population confronts us with a problem of such catastrophic proportions that we could be forgiven for applying desperate remedies, or at least taking a few risks to preserve some sort of demographic balance, though this, one can be sure, is not the reason why most women take the pill.

Whatever the advocates of the pill may say, there are side-effects – some rare, some common, some serious, some trivial. The question is, can we afford to ignore them? And the question has been there since the day in May 1960 when the US Food and Drug Administration first sanctioned the general prescription of 'Enovid' for contraceptive purposes. The 'birth pill' was an experiment then: nobody knew what the long-term effects would be. Nobody knows now.

Ehrlich, the inventor of 'Salvarsan', the first truly specific drug – against syphilis – was trying to find a 'magic bullet' against disease, a chemical which would zero in to its precise target and knock out the offending organism, a drug as accurate as an air-to-ground missile which would work quickly, cleanly and without waste against the syphilis microbe.

This has remained the pharmacologist's ideal. The pill could hardly be more different. It is not a magic bullet so much as a blast of grapeshot, an indiscriminate agent which not only smothers its target organs but spreads its effects to others, too. In the comparatively massive doses in which it was first used, it has been described as a type of pharmacological overkill, a fine example of blunderbuss therapy – except that it is not therapy at all, because women who take the pill are not ill. It is unlike any other drug in the history of medicine.

Its uniqueness lies not only in its place in the history of pharmaceutics. The pill is also helping to overturn conventional ideas of sexual morality, and, coming as it did at a time of increasing sexual liberty, it arrived almost exactly on cue. And whereas history suggests that periods of sexual licence tend to alternate with periods of greater restraint, it is doubtful whether the pendulum could ever swing back again now that, in the West at least, women's sexual emancipation is virtually complete.

Virtually complete, rather than absolute, because the question of safety still remains. If the pill is not medically safe, or, to make an important distinction, not safe enough, its usefulness as an emancipating force is impaired. It is not necessarily ruined. As the recent history of cigarette-smoking has shown, men and women can easily ignore a long-term danger while they enjoy a short-term reward.

From many points of view the pill is a major medico-social advance, but it is only the first step. No doubt future generations, looking back on the nineteen-sixties, will be amazed that we were prepared to stomach a pharmaceutical product of such uncertain effect to further our comfort and convenience. But the notion of systemic contraception, contraception from within, is certain to be salvaged from our first fumbling attempt to make pregnancy a matter of choice rather than chance. Some may doubt if we ever shall find the answer. Dr Celso-Ramon Garcia, one of the first doctors to work on the original formulation of the pill said to me: 'I have never claimed that the pill is the ideal contraceptive. There can never be an ideal contraceptive. Not unless you believe in Utopia.'

Men may smugly consider that they have extended our power over the environment, but nature has a way of pulling the carpet from under the scientists' feet. It seems to be the fate of mankind never to score a total victory over the natural circumstances to which we are born: or to put it less grandly, nature is not easily fooled.

Meanwhile, without always knowing it, those twenty million women have been taking part in both an experiment and a gamble. But the stakes are high, and the time available is short. As Francis Bacon wrote, 'Nature is a labyrinth, in which the very haste you move with will make you lose your way.'

# 1. Something in Never-never Land

'PILL ... *A small ball of medicinal substance, of a size convenient to be swallowed whole*' –
Shorter Oxford English Dictionary

'*Was the pill discovered or was it invented? That's quite a question. Quite a question*' –
American research chemist

Scientific discoveries do not always happen in life as they do in fiction. The drama is usually lacking, and there is hardly ever a single moment of enlightenment which can be hailed later on, still less at the time, as the blinding revelation which belongs to scientific history.

Nobody cried '*Eureka!*' when the first contraceptive pill in the world was held aloft in a pair of laboratory tweezers. Nobody made a speech, nobody opened the champagne. This was not the Great Moment in the story of the pill, and there really are no great moments, only a succession of bright ideas which gradually began to add up, and over the years could be seen to point to a specific object – the control of conception by a tablet.

But people like to think of the progress of science as punctuated by astonishing incidents happening to remarkable men. Several versions of the story of how the oral contraceptive came about include an account of a night in the early nineteen-fifties when one man made the kind of discovery which is generally expected of scientists. On a night of tension, it has been recorded, a confrontation took place in New York. Mrs Margaret Sanger, the birth control pioneer, in the name of womanhood entreated the late Dr Gregory Pincus the research biologist, to rally the world of science in a now-or-never effort to find a new approach to contraception. Pincus, it is said, silent and concerned drove back alone to Shrewsbury, Massachusetts, and on the road the truth struck him like a thunderbolt : a contraceptive pill swallowed like an aspirin! By Jupiter, one can almost hear him say, it might just work . . .

A different version, of what could be the same incident, is told by Pincus's widow, Elizabeth Pincus. It, too, has its share of drama. Margaret Sanger, says Mrs Pincus, brought to her husband's office a Mrs Stanley McCormick, a widow with a great deal of money. Together, the two women urged Pincus to find at all costs a contraceptive pill, and fast. He thought about the problem, and with a snap of the fingers knew exactly where to go to find the answer, or at least the beginning of the answer : a footnote nobody else remembered in a scientific article nearly twenty years earlier, which had shown that the sex hormone progesterone would prevent female rabbits from releasing an ovum.

Elizabeth Pincus recounts: 'When he finally told me, he said, "Lizuska, I've got it." I said, "What have you got?" He said, "I think we have a contraceptive pill." I said, "My God, why didn't you *tell* me?" Then he told me. Exactly. I said, "Look, when these women asked you to produce a contraceptive pill, this was a fantasy. These were bright, intelligent women but they wanted something in never-never land. Did you think you could ever *get* the pill?" He said, "Lizuska, everything is possible in science."'

Not only does memory play the fool with facts, but the temptation to rewrite those key scenes and give them in retrospect the kind of production they ought to have had is hard to resist. Instead of the disillusionments, false starts and red herrings which the work actually entailed, posterity can enjoy a moment of discovery, part-real, part-invented, with its outlines sharpened and all the doubts and qualifications flattened out.

New pharmaceutical products happen in two ways: either by accident, or because someone took a deliberate decision to create a particular drug for a particular purpose. Penicillin is an example of the first. The story of how Fleming happened to notice something unusual about one of his cultures, which had been affected by something that blew in through the window from Praed Street, is one of the best-known incidents in modern medicine. The drug industry could tell of dozens more, less momentous than that: often by-products emerge from one piece of research in the shape of new formulations which were not what the chemists were looking for, but which turn out to have applications in some different medical situation.

Of the second type of drug – the tailor-made, custom-built pharmaceutical devised for one specific reason – the best example is probably the oral contraceptive. Or rather, not the pill itself but the so-called 'progestational' synthetic agent which was its starting-point. It was not devised as an oral contraceptive, but as a man-made substitute for the natural hormone progesterone: unlike the natural product, it could be swallowed and would still work.

As luck would have it, synthetic progesterone came at exactly the right moment, when injections of the natural hormone were already being tried as a means of preventing women from ovulating. Gregory Pincus and his collaborators needed a better way of doing this than pumping in large doses of natural progesterone. And now the synthetic versions, the 'progestogens' or 'progestins', were providentially at hand to supply the answer. Pincus could not have launched the first trials of an oral contraceptive unless the orally effective progestogens had been developed, in the laboratories of two drug companies, G. D. Searle and Syntex. The progestogens themselves could not have been developed had it not been for the synthesis of natural progesterone, in the previous decade, by the chemist Russell Marker. Marker would not have synthesized progesterone had it not been for the gathering interest in the hormone as a method of treating gynaecological disorders.

Two separate movements combined to produce the first contraceptive pills. One was this rapid series of advances in organic chemistry which took place over a period of some fifteen years. The other was the growing need for a new form of contraceptive which was more reliable than existing methods and which could provide some way of keeping back the headlong increase in world population. But the idea of 'oral contraception' had been in the air for some time before Pincus started working on the problem in the nineteen-fifties. It had been known for some time that ovulation – the monthly release of an egg ready for fertilization – could be prevented by hormone injections, and so it was clear that somewhere along these lines there could lie the solution to the problem of finding a contraceptive which worked, as it were, from within the body.

What is now disarmingly called the 'classical' contraceptive pill contains synthetic versions of two natural hormones, progesterone and oestrogen. Both are secreted in women's ovaries during certain phases of the menstrual cycle. Oestrogen is produced in a crescendo, starting during the period of menstrual flow and for the following two weeks or so, after which it tails off. The word, of fairly recent coinage, means literally producing a state of sexual readiness (or being 'on heat'), and the function of the hormone is to prepare the woman's body for conception and pregnancy. Progesterone, on the other hand, is produced for about ten days before menstrual flow begins, and it originates in a gland called the corpus luteum ('yellow body'), formed at the site where the egg broke away to travel down to the womb.

For many years it had been realized that this progesterone-producing gland had some role in preventing the release of another egg during the same month. In the eighteen-nineties a Viennese gynaecologist, Emil Knauer, demonstrated that a hormone existed in the ovary : he transplanted ovaries into animals which had none of their own (they had either been castrated or were too young), and found that the animals developed sex characteristics. In fact the word hormone did not yet exist: it was coined in 1905 by a classicist-friend for the benefit of the endocrinologist Ernest Starling, to describe chemical messengers, which were secreted in the glands and carried to target organs to produce a specific effect.

Over the next twenty years, experiments with animals showed that once the corpus luteum was functioning, the animal would not ovulate again until the next reproductive cycle. But in 1921 the idea of oral contraception reached print, based on these experiments with the sex-glands of animals. An Austrian Professor, Ludwig Haberlandt, had done another transplant experiment in his laboratory at Innsbruck. He put the ovaries of pregnant rabbits and guinea-pigs into animals which were not pregnant. The animals became temporarily sterile. He called it a 'sterilization method'. And he added that since current methods of contraception were unreliable, something similar could perhaps be applied to women who did not want any more children. He went on with the almost clairvoyant observation that possibly extracts from the ovaries of pregnant animals might be taken by mouth.

Oral contraception was on record, but it was hardly more than a theoretical possibility. What the substances were which had to be taken to achieve contraception this way, and whether they *could* be taken by mouth, were other questions again.

The answers to both of them became clearer not long afterwards, when the first sex hormone was isolated. It was oestrogen, or more specifically one of the oestrogens, which are now known to number at least twenty. As other substances in the oestrogen family were isolated, it began to be possible to see what their effects might be when used as drugs. It was found that if women who suffered from dysmenorrhoea (painful periods) were given oestrogen, they had less pain – and also, they would not ovulate.

Progesterone too was isolated, from sow's ovaries, and was shortly afterwards shown to inhibit the sexual cycle in rats. More significant was a paper published in 1937 by three research scientists from Pennsylvania University; it was this paper, as we shall see, which was to form the basis for Pincus's experiments, for the three men had described the effect of giving progesterone to rabbits. Unlike women, female rabbits only ovulate when they have mated. The rabbits in the Pennsylvania experiment had been mated. But they did not ovulate.

Similar results came from giving progesterone to a succession of different species, and it occurred to one research worker that the progesterone was having an effect similar to pregnancy, when ovulation was also inhibited. A gynaecologist at Columbia University, Raphael Kurzrok, pointed out that sometimes perfectly healthy women failed to ovulate. The corpus luteum therefore did not form, and consequently there was no progesterone in circulation. The usual sequel to the production of progesterone was that the lining of the womb became thicker, stronger, and able to make a hospitable nest for the ovum if it should be fertilized – but none of this took place in the absence of progesterone. Monthly cycles with no ovulation, Kurzrok remarked, were typical of the time when a woman is breast-feeding. 'If such cycles should be produced at will,' he said, 'we would have available a safe contraceptive method.' The other ovarian hormone, oestrogen, offered similar possibilities. It too would prevent or delay ovulation. So it might be possible to make a woman temporarily infertile by giving her oestrogen.

Gradually the possibilities of chemical control of conception were unfolding, and by 1945 Professor Fuller Albright of Harvard, for one, had a prophetically clear idea of the potentialities of, as he called it, 'birth control by hormone therapy'. 'Since preventing ovulation prevents pregnancy,' he wrote, 'one could employ the same principles in birth control as in preventing dysmenororrhoea.' One could use one of the newly discovered synthetic oestrogens, stilboestrol. Said Albright: 'Thus, for example, if an individual took l-mg of diethylstilboestrol by mouth daily from the first day of her period for the next six weeks, she would not ovulate during this interval; if she then still wanted to continue the birth control further, she could continue the stilboestrol and take a course of progesterone to cause menstruation.' It would be like stretching the normal menstrual period to nearly double its length, or longer if need be, and doing it according to the natural sequence of hormones: circulating oestrogen followed by a shorter period of circulating progesterone. Straightaway all kinds of advantages began to suggest themselves. 'One could juggle the above therapeutics,' Albright suggested, 'to make the menstrual period come on the least undesirable day.'

Unfortunately, the prospect of 'periods on demand' outlined by Albright was a distant one for the time being. The fact was that the 'therapeutics' which had to be juggled with simply did not exist in a form which would make daily doses of selected hormones available for more than a few women.

The hormones were manufactured from such sources as human urine, stallions' urine, bulls' testicles and sows' ovaries. The need for elaborate production processes made supplies of oestrogen and progesterone both scarce and expensive. It was a frustrating situation, because doctors wanted to extend their knowledge of how these hormones could be used medicinally, and the more that was known about them the greater the demand became. Oestrogen was required for treating women whose periods were painful or irregular; progesterone, for women who were 'habitual aborters', whose own supply of the hormone was inadequate to maintain a pregnancy.

What was needed was some cheap and convenient way of manufacturing these sought-after substances which would make their laborious production from animal sources a thing of the past. It was around this time that Russell E. Marker entered the story.

Marker, Professor of Organic Chemistry at State College, Pennsylvania, was an extraordinary person: touchy, difficult and erratic, but an exteremely clever chemist. Though he had been appointed to his professorship at Pennsylvania at thirty-two, he had never taken a doctorate. He had finished the work for it, but never submitted his thesis because of an argument with the head of his department at the University of Maryland, which is said to have culminated in Marker's tearing up the work before his professor's eyes. In spite of this unpromising beginning, Marker found a job at the Rockefeller Institute for Medical Research, where his work on the microscopic structure of organic compounds began to make his name known. This job, too, ended in a quarrel. Marker walked out, and shortly afterwards took the chair of Organic Chemistry at State College.

With financial backing from Parke, Davis and Co, the drug firm, Marker there produced a continuous flow of scientific papers dealing with the chemistry of steroids, an important group of natural substances, which run into many thousands. The steroids in the human body include the sex hormones. Many of Marker's papers on these compounds led directly to lucrative new production processes for the fine chemicals used to make drugs and medicines.

All in all the problem of finding a new and simpler starting-point for the commercial manufacture of sex hormones was very much in Marker's line. He made a start on it in 1939. The best source, he thought, was a substance called sapogenin, which has a chemical resemblance to the steroids (and which, as it happens, is used as a foam stabilizer in some kinds of contraceptive tablet).

The structure of sapogenin, when analysed in the chemical laboratory, can be seen to include a long pendulous 'side-chain', rather like a tail, attached to the four rings of the molecule. In this respect it is like cholesterol, the fatty substance which the body itself uses as a starting-point for making steroids. To make steroids such as progesterone out of cholesterol, the side-chain has to be removed by chemical reactions, and this the body can accomplish without difficulty; but it is very much harder for chemists to repeat the process. So Marker's problem was to find a way of dismantling the side-chain from sapogenin and making it resemble progesterone.

The first thing was to find out what the side-chain consisted of. This had never been done before, but Marker managed to do it, and find a way of removing it from the molecule, all within a few months. The sapogenin he used was taken from the root of the sarsaparilla plant, and it was called sarsapogenin. This he was able to convert into progesterone, and by further chemical juggling into the male hormone testosterone.

This was not the end of the affair, however, because the yield of progesterone from sarsapogenin was too small to have any commercial value. But there was a possibility that other plants of the sarsaparilla family might produce a far higher yield of sapogenin. The most likely place to find them was in the sub-tropical south-west of the United States and in Mexico. So Marker spent his summer vacation in 1940 searching for plants which might contain the substance he needed. He also enlisted the help of botanists he met on his travels and asked them to send him any plants which might conceivably be a source.

Soon, parcels of obscure and malodorous plants were arriving at State College. Nearly five tons of tropical greenery accumulated in Marker's laboratory, where he and his students proceeded to take them apart chemically. Many yielded no sapogenin at all. But many others did produce sapogenins previously unknown to botanic chemistry and Marker gave them whimsical names. One was called Kammogenin, after the research director of Parke, Davis, another was called Rockogenin after a University colleague nicknamed Rocky. One supposed sapogenin turned out to be an artifact – an unwanted substance, a kind of cuckoo in the nest that had intruded during the chemical processing. Marker got his revenge on a rival by calling it after him, Fiesergenin.

Of all the varieties of weird plant he collected, one produced the highest yield of all. It was a plant found in Mexico and known there as *cabeza de negro*. Its proper name was dioscorea, and it was a species of wild yam – the potato of the tropical and subtropical countries. Marker considered that diosgenin, as he called it, was the solution to his problem, and for that matter to that of the pharmaceutical industry: a cheap and abundant source of supply for a synthetic progesterone.

Progesterone at that time was selling at around £25 a gramme. It was obvious to Marker that a source of synthetic progesterone would make a lot of money. So the equally obvious thing, to him at least, was for someone to put capital into producing progesterone from diosgenin and selling it on a commercial basis, preferably near the source of supply. But now his troubles began again. No one could see things his way. There was a war on. This was not the moment to lay out capital on such a precarious adventure. Besides, Mexico in the nineteen-forties was not everyone's idea of a convenient location for the manufacture of fine chemicals. The Mexican pharmaceutical industry was virtually non-existent: there were no facilities for processing the black root, and what was more the *cabeza de negro* was hardly the most accessible source material, for it grew in steamy, hilly jungle where nobody in his senses ever went. And was Mexico politically stable? How could any large company setting up an establishment there be sure of the future?

Even hunting in the jungle for the right plant seemed easy compared with raising money to back his hunch. Marker found. 'Nobody would help me,' he recalled recently. 'I tried all over, I even showed them what yield I'd got. They said it was impossible. There was no equipment, no chemical industry in Mexico. Everyone predicted it would be a failure.'

The obvious source of funds was the drug industry. No sale: the scheme was not practical. His own college, predictably, proved no more enthusiastic. Financing the manufacture of synthetic hormones seemed to them tangential to the proper occupation of a Pennsylvania academic institution. Marker decided to go it alone. Once again he staged an abrupt exit. In mid-term he walked out of State College and took himself off, alone and with hardly any money, to Mexico City. There he rented a small house in a back street; behind it was a stable which had been used as a potter's shed, and was empty except, luckily, for a few mules. Marker conscripted them, and set off into the mountains, like a character in a B. Traven novel, a short, stocky, bald figure smoking a cigar. Talking about it recently, he dismissed the whole thing as 'not too difficult'. He added, 'It was kind of an interesting vacation.' But surely the country was difficult? 'Well, I certainly didn't run into any Americans down there,' Marker said mildly. 'It was Indian country, mostly. But I thought I'd find something. I expected to get some result.'

He was right. Within a matter of months he had brought back by mule some two dozen sacks of dioscorea root, and, working in his shed with improvised equipment, he had made a sizeable quantity of progesterone.

In 1943 he walked into the offices of a small pharmaceutical wholesale firm in Mexico City, Laboratorios Hormona, run by two European émigrés, Dr Emeric Somlo, a Hungarian, and Dr Federico Lehmann, a German. In his hand Marker carried two pickle-jars wrapped in newspaper: did they want any progesterone? He unwrapped his parcel and revealed to the amazed businessmen two jars filled to the brim with white powder – 4½lb of progesterone made from disgenin, enough to fetch some £45,000 at the current price.

The upshot of this confrontation was that Marker was invited to join Somlo and Lehmann in a new company, formed specifically to market the synthetic hormone. The company was incorporated in Mexico City on 21 January 1944, under the name of Syntex S.A.

Nevertheless, placing Marker's technique on a regular footing did not exactly open the flood-gates of production. The new company was still only a small one and loomed insignificantly, if at all, in an industry then on the threshold of a breathtaking period of expansion. During the first year of Syntex's operations, only a few more pounds of the precious chemical were manufactured, though even this was enough to send a warning tremor through those sections of the pharmaceutical industry concerned with hormone products. Potentially, Syntex was in a strong position, with the demand for progesterone going up continually, for treating irregular or painful periods. But in time to ruin any complacent feelings Somlo and Lehmann may have entertained, relations between them and Marker became strained. There was a final, sharp disagreement. And in 1945 Marker walked out as abruptly as he had marched off the campus of Pennsylvania State or appeared in the doorway of Laboratorios Hormona. This time, he took with him the notes of his laboratory process, and also, according to one story, switched labels on his storage jars as a kind of booby-trap for anyone taking his place at the bench.

For a short while Marker concerned himself with other pharmaceutical ventures, but it appears that he had suddenly tired of chemistry altogether. There followed a period of some twenty years in which he had to all intents and purposes disappeared. Was he dead? No one knew, including former colleagues and friends. Letters sent to him at his usual address came back marked 'Gone Away'. Then he reappeared suddenly at his old hotel in Mexico City – and found himself, apparently to his surprise, hailed as the father of today's flourishing Mexican hormone industry. He now divides his time, once again, between Mexico City and the town of State College, with occasional trips to Europe. He is busy collecting not plant seeds but reproductions of famous pieces of silver. He has a large collection and they are made specially for him by Mexican silversmiths. Letters to him elicit courteous, but only mildly interested replies: he has retired from scientific work, he says, has not kept up with modern developments in the steroid hormones and has never been interested in their medicinal or contraceptive uses.

Marker and Syntex now speak of each other in cordial and respectful terms. Apart from what he did for Mexican chemistry (and the country's economy) he is also enthusiastically praised for – in the words of Carl Djerassi – his 'monumental contribution' to chemical research. 'I think,' says Djerassi, who is Vice-President of Syntex Research, 'he deserves the Nobel Prize.'

Marker's reputation at Syntex cannot have been so exalted in 1945, for without him production of progesterone ground to a halt. There ensued a hasty search to find someone who could take over where Marker had left off, and in a Havana drug firm, Somlo found a fellow Hungarian, Dr George Rosenkranz, who seemed to fit the bill. Rosenkranz had worked on steroid chemistry in Switzerland, followed Marker's publications on the subject and even succeeded in making both progesterone and testosterone, the principal male sex hormone, using Mexican sarsaparilla. Within a few days, in a virtuoso display of chemical technique, Rosenkranz had reconstructed Marker's synthetic process, and he swiftly set Syntex's production back on its feet. He then proceeded to synthesize testosterone, together with an important hormone produced by the adrenal gland, desoxycorticosterone. His starting-point in each case was diosgenin.

Next came the oestrogens. Oestrone and oestradiol were synthesized, from diosgenin again, by Carl Djerassi. By the early fifties Syntex had become the major supplier of synthetic hormones to drug houses in Europe and America, and the use of these products to treat patients whose natural supply was deficient had gained momentum. In 1954 Syntex delivered one ton of progesterone to one single company. Prices had fallen precipitously: progesterone was now worth less than £1 per gramme.

But there was another problem for the chemists to overcome. Synthetic progesterone shared a serious disadvantage with the natural variety: it was ineffective when it was taken by mouth. If it was to do any good it had to be taken by injection, sometimes in large and uncomfortable doses. The objective of a hormone product which could be swallowed as pill or potion, as foreseen by Fuller Albright in 1945 and, more remotely, by Haberlandt in 1921, remained elusive.

On the other hand a substantial clue had come from a report given by a chemistry professor at the University of Pennsylvania, Professor Max Ehrenstein, to an American Chemical Society meeting in Cleveland in April 1944. He had shown that, contrary to the usual belief, one could change the structure of progesterone and yet not change its effects. If this were so, it was possible that one could alter the structure of progesterone to make it effective when swallowed, yet not diminish its potency. Ehrenstein had simplified the chemistry of a progesterone-like steroid, called strophanthidin, ending with a crude, resinous material which he then proceeded to test on rabbits: it had the same activity as progesterone in causing changes to the lining of the womb. But once again the research stagnated, interest petered out, and no more progress had been made by the time Carl Djerassi arrived at Syntex in Mexico City in 1949.

With over 650 scientific publications to his credit, including six books, Djerassi is a man of powerful intellect and understandably one of the Syntex Corporation's favourite sons. A cultivated man now in his late forties (he was born in Vienna in 1923), he attends Pugwash conferences and, as well as being Vice-President of Syntex Research at Palo Alto, he is also Professor of Chemistry at Stanford University; he is driven the couple of miles between the two establishments in a company limousine.

Djerassi was the man who, in 1950, tackled the problem of creating synthetic progesterone that could be taken by mouth, the step that was to lead directly to the formulation of the contraceptive pill. He followed the lead suggested in Ehrenstein's experiment, making structural changes similar to those

Ehrenstein had made, but using as a basis a compound derived from diosgenin. It proved a relatively easy matter to make the changes he wanted, and when the resulting substance was given by injection it turned out to have somewhere between four and eight times the potency of the natural hormone.

But although this was encouraging, it still had not produced a progesterone-like substance that worked by mouth. So Djerassi took another steroid, related to the male sex hormone testosterone. It was known to be effective to some extent as a progestational agent when swallowed – though a dose six times greater was required than when it was injected. But it seemed possible that if the same structural changes were made to this new steroid, it might be both active when swallowed, and a potent progestogen.

In late 1951 Djerassi went through seven separate chemical processes, at the end of which an entirely new molecule emerged. Its full-dress name was 19-nor-17-alpha-ethinyltestosterone – or, for short, norethisterone. His prediction was amply confirmed: it had 'a high order of potency,' Djerassi reported, and it had the required effect when it was swallowed.

Djerassi at Syntex was not, however, the only one to become interested in the possibilities originally suggested in Ehrenstein's report. In Chicago, Illinois, research chemists at the drug firm of G. D. Searle & Co also began to look for a way of making an orally effective synthetic progesterone. And their version, closely similar to norethisterone, was patented shortly afterwards under the name norethynodrel. Now that the compounds existed, the next problem was to find a use for them: that, as it will appear, did not cause much difficulty, for already Pincus, in Shrewsbury, Massachusetts, had started work on the suppression of ovulation by means of progesterone.

It has been argued that the chemists' contribution to the development of the contraceptive pill – which was now a logical step from what had been achieved in the laboratory – has been underrated. The people who argue this are, of course, the chemists themselves, but there is some truth in their complaint. Organic chemistry is a complicated subject, with its cumbersome names and its preoccupation with the structure of com-

plex chemicals. It is far easier to appreciate the enterprise of
the doctor who first successfully uses the weapon which the
chemists put into his hands. In the case of the progestogens,
the people who took the final step of using them for contraceptive purposes were the ones who collected the honours. Yet
the creation of the progestogens is in some ways an object
lesson in the devising of a new pharmaceutical drug. They did
not emerge by accident. They were not some unexpected bonus
from research ostensibly heading in a different direction. They
were not laboratory mistakes. Instead, the chemists set themselves a specific problem. Solving it meant having to work out
relationships between the minute features of a chemical configuration and the effects of that configuration. When this had
been done, the work was brought to the appropriate conclusion: the creation of a chemical not found in nature, and con-
structed to have the effect planned for it.

But it is just at this point of success that the trouble with the
pill begins. The progestogens, and the oestrogenic compounds
which are their partners in the 'classical' oral contraceptive,
are not natural products. They are synthetic adaptations of
natural products, in which subtle variations have been made to
obtain the desired result. On paper, the variations have a way
of appearing trivial. But they may be gross differences when
applied continuously to the intricate machinery of the human
body – machinery too ingenious for chemists to duplicate, far
too sensitive to be misled by even the smallest molecular variation.

# 2. The Road to Shrewsbury

'*Whenever I get discouraged with the current situation I look back over the last decade or two and I cannot help but be thrilled by the vast progress that has been made. Then, the future appears very bright*' –

Dr Alan Guttmacher, 'Babies by Choice or by Chance', 1960

'*Once when I was feeling depressed and thinking, "Oh God, it's all too much," I said, "Goody, let's go out and let's get a cart and we'll sell lemons, it is just not worth it." He said, "Stick with me kid, and you'll be wearing diamonds . . ."*' –

Mrs Gregory Pincus, 1969

Carl Djerassi's report of the synthesis of his progesterone-like compound was given in Milwaukee in April 1952, at a meeting of the American Chemical Society. In due course it reached print under the names of Djerassi and three Syntex colleagues, Luis Miramontes, George Rosenkranz and Franz Sondheimer. It was a technical paper, barely penetrable for anyone but an analytical chemist, a laboratory report from specialists to fellow-specialists, and, for a piece of work with such far-reaching consequences, would strike the outsider as disappointingly low-key.

In substance, the results meant that doctors were furnished with a new and powerful compound rich in its implications for medicine: a synthetic drug which would do the things natural progesterone would do – and it could be taken by mouth. A new word was needed to describe the man-made 'progestational' substances: they were progestogens, or progestins.

By the time Djerassi's paper appeared in its final form the new drug norethisterone (norethindrone in the USA) had been tried out. The first creatures to be given it were rabbits. The first doctor to administer it was someone who had been involved with the subject for some time. He had assisted Max Ehrenstein in his work on the original crude 19-norprogesterone made from strophanthidin. His name was Dr Roy Hertz and he was working at the National Institutes of Health at Bethesda, outside Washington. He was to play a rather different role in the later history of oral contraception.

Djerassi sent Hertz some of the new synthetic substance – not the oily mixture created by Ehrenstein, but a pure crystalline powder. Hertz found the Syntex product between four and eight times more effective than natural progesterone when it was taken by mouth, judging by the drug's action on the lining of the womb, where the cells proliferated as though to create the appropriate environment for a fertilized egg.

Hertz went on to other animals: guinea-pigs, monkeys – and then human beings. In the first trials on human patients norethisterone was used in the way that natural progesterone would be used, except that less of it was needed. Women whose gynaecological problems arose from a supposed deficiency of progesterone were given the new synthetic drug to correct the faulty balance of hormones. The first women to have the treatment were three patients of Hertz's at Bethesda, in the Clinical Centre of the National Institute of Child Health and Human Development. They received doses of between five and ten milligrammes, strictly in an attempt to control menstrual irregularities, which they did. There was no question of using it to prevent pregnancy.

However, though the Syntex people may have been first in the field with an oral progestogen, they were about to have the ground, or part of it, cut from under their feet. Djerassi's report to the American Chemical Society was printed in full in the Society's *Journal* in April 1954. In November of the following year a patent was applied for at the US Patent Office in the name of Dr F. B. Colton, a biochemist working with the pharmaceutical company G. D. Searle, of Illinois. It was a patent for another synthetic steroid, different from the product described in Djerassi's paper, a patent for which had been sought by Syntex at the earliest opportunity, in 1951. When the chemical maps of the two molecules, Searle's and Syntex's, are compared,

it takes some time for an untrained eye to spot the difference, which rests on the position of a double bond, or link,
between two of the carbon atoms. The processes involved in
synthesizing the Searle steroid are closely related to those in
Djerassi's account. No theoretical papers had appeared from
Searle's research staff in advance of the patent application, and
when one queries the comparative suddenness of their arrival
on the scene, Searle's point stonily to US patent number
2,725,389, in the name of Dr Frank B. Colton.

According to Searle's own account, from about 1951 onwards
a group of chemists at the company's laboratories had been
searching for progestational compounds which could be swallowed. Dr Colton was one of the team, and had followed up,
independently, it is implied, the clue supplied by Ehrenstein and
his strophanthidin. 'A whole series' of 19-nor steroids, Searle's
have said, was tested by the company, until in 1952 a compound with the code name SC-4642 duly became the subject of
the Colton patent.

Taken at face value, the two accounts add up to, at the least,
a startling coincidence: two groups of pharmaceutical chemists
arrived independently at almost the identical solution. It is not
impossible, though it does sound unlikely. And no suit for
patent infringement was ever filed by Syntex, though there are
hints that such a thing was contemplated. Searle officials coolly
describe the company as 'the inventors of the Pill' and there
was even a plan at one time for the words 'The Pill' to be copy-
righted in Searle's name. The company's 'corporate policy
counsellor' James W. Irwin recently explained, 'It was never
tried. We toyed with the idea. After all, if you could patent the
word "Coke" for Coca-Cola why not "The Pill" for the oral
contraceptive? So we kicked the idea around. But we never
took any action.'

For some time before all this took place, Searle had been re-
taining as consultant in biological research the services of Dr
Gregory Goodman Pincus. Though he was not concerned with
the development work with Colton, he was shortly to become
deeply involved in synthetic steroids – and the creation of the
pill.

Pincus's base was a private research establishment in Shrewsbury, Massachusetts, with a staff of around twenty, but grandly called the Worcester Foundation for Experimental Biology. With Dr Hudson Hoagland (now its President), Pincus had started the foundation in 1944. He had already made a name for himself in endocrinology and was the organizer of the annual Laurentian Hormone Conference. The son of Russian-Jewish parents, he had been born in Woodbine, New Jersey, in 1903, had graduated in science at Cornell and then gone on to Harvard to take a master's degree and a doctorate of science. He had also travelled and worked abroad: once, during the twenties, at the Kaiser Wilhelm Institute in Berlin, and for two separate spells at Cambridge University.

At first his subject was nominally agriculture. But quite early on he developed an interest in genetics and the study of inherited characteristics. The reason for this, according to his Chinese *émigré* associate at the Worcester Foundation, Dr Min-Chueh Chang, was that Pincus himself had an inherited defect, though a minor one: he was colour blind. Like many colour blind people his eyesight was unusually sharp, says Chang, who claims that Pincus told him he could spot a four-leaf clover while walking through a field. Pincus had also had the luck to be born with a photographic memory, and could read a book at three times the speed of a normal person (he preferred crime novels, one a night).

From genetics to embryology and the study of reproduction was not a mighty step, and Pincus became more and more interested in the mechanism of fertilization: how sperm penetrates the egg, what it needs to make the event possible, how the egg is induced to descend to the Fallopian tubes from the ovary, why, when once fertilized, it beds down in the womb – the whole obscure and intriguing business of how mammals reproduce themselves. Much of his work was original, ingenious, and highly regarded. One of his achievements was to induce in the laboratory the maturation processes that occur in the rabbit egg before it has been fertilized. But, in his thirties, his career had a bad set-back. He announced that he had also made a rabbit egg develop without benefit of fertilization: a dramatic demonstration, if true, of the elusive phenomenon of virgin birth. But no one was able to repeat the experiment. Pincus's stock slumped. Yet the error, which might have disgraced a less resilient man, was forgotten.

From this and similar lines of inquiry he drew a series of conclusions not only about the hormones involved in reproduction, but where it might be possible to step in and influence the course of events from outside. Fertilization of an ovum was, as he put it, 'not merely a chance meeting of egg and sperm'. It was an event that could not happen unless the sperm were mature and had undergone the process called capacitation. Nor could it happen unless the egg itself were ready for it. He realized that the follicle, the structure in the ovary that produces the egg, does so because it is set going by hormones produced in the pituitary, the pea-sized gland in the base of the skull. Something he did not then appreciate was that, if too great a quantity of the ovarian hormones was at large in the body, this would prevent the pituitary hormones from being produced, thus undoing the 'feedback' principle which sees to it that the body's internal balance of hormones is retained. This would be one of the central points of dispute when the pill was finally produced.

But his conclusions all pointed, he said, to the possibility that fertility, and so pregnancy, might be controllable – by 'manipulating' the egg's environment. And, in particular, manipulating the hormones which controlled that environment.

Even so it was not until after the war, during which Pincus worked on the relation of hormones to physical and mental stress, that he started on work which would take these ideas further.

As we have seen, the event that set him off was the meeting that occurred in 1951 with Margaret Sanger. The way it has been described has conferred on the meeting a portentousness it almost certainly does not merit. According to what can almost be described as legend, Pincus was summoned to New York, ostensibly to spend the evening with an old friend, Dr Abraham Stone. There too was Mrs Sanger, the sixty-eight-year old heroine of the American birth control movement, organizer of international birth control conferences, founder of the International Planned Parenthood Federation, writer, publisher and even one-time hawker of broadsheets, pamphlets and books explaining the ABC of family planning. She had survived ridicule, public odium, jail, pelting with rotten fruit and the organized persecution of the puritan wing whose views were nicely summed up by the anonymous senator who declared, 'If I were the Creator and were making the universe all over again, I would leave sex out.'

An indomitable fighter for women's rights, Margaret Sanger had lived to see a profound change in people's acceptance of birth control. In the eighteen-eighties, when she was born, the New York Society for the Suppression of Vice, under the leadership of Anthony Comstock, the Post Office Inspector and scourge of the sensual man, was in full cry against birth control and free thought, being responsible in a space of ten years, notes Peter Fryer in *The Birth Controllers*, for 700 arrests, 333 sentences of imprisonment totalling 155 years and 13 days, fines totalling $65,256 and the confiscation of 27,856 lb of 'obscene books and 64,836 'articles for immoral use, of rubber, etc.'. By the end of Margaret Sanger's life – she died in 1966 – what had come to be called 'Comstockery' was finished for good, and she had been responsible as much as any other single person for bringing the change about. But at the time of her meeting with Pincus, she believed the campaign for easier contraception was losing impetus, because of the inadequacy of the contraceptives available. With the world population increase beginning to assume alarming proportions, the time was ripe for some entirely new approach that would make coitus interruptus, the dutch cap and the condom seem antique and outmoded.

Margaret Sanger was confident that a breakthrough was to come from the research scientists. A modern method of birth control should draw on modern knowledge of reproductive physiology. Maybe Dr Pincus was the man. As we have seen, the story goes that Pincus succumbed to Mrs Sanger's persuasion and left New York next day with the promise of $2,100 to cover the expenses of the first year's investigation. On the road back to Shrewsbury, 'he analysed the problem with quick and incisive clarity', runs one account, arriving back at the Foundation 180 miles away with the fully-fledged idea that progesterone was the answer. It worked in rabbits, as the Pennsylvania research of 1937 had shown: why not in women too? A woman's body produces large quantities of progesterone during pregnancy: *ergo* progesterone, the 'pregnancy hormone' would, if taken at other times, prevent ovulation just as if the woman were pregnant. In fact there was nothing very original in this observation: the problem was how to make use of it to produce some practical, everyday chemical contraceptive.

In his own account of the beginning of his research on contraception, Pincus does not refer to any meeting in New York, but to a visit *from* Margaret Sanger in 1951 as one of the two 'overtly ascertainable factors' which set the research moving in Shrewsbury (the other being 'the emergence of the appreciation of the importance of the "population explosion"').

Either on that or on some other occasion, Margaret Sanger was accompanied by another woman, Mrs Stanley McCormick, whose contribution was in some ways much more important.

Mrs McCormick, who died in 1967, aged ninety-two, was very rich indeed. She was also, according to Gregory Pincus's widow, not a woman to be trifled with: 'Insignificant nothing, she was tall and carried herself like a ramrod. Little old woman she was *not*. She was a grenadier.'

Mrs McCormick was also one of the first women to graduate from the Massachusetts Institute of Technology, and like Margaret Sanger a long-time supporter of women's rights – including the right to practise birth control. Katharine McCormick's father-in-law, Cyrus McCormick, inventor of the mechanical reaper, had made a fortune out of farm machinery, and a substantial part of the money was now at Mrs McCormick's disposal. She herself was childless. Dr John Rock, the Boston physician who was to join forces with Pincus later in the research, says of her : 'She was as rich as *Croesus*. She had a *vast* fortune. Her lawyer told me she couldn't even spend the interest on her *interest*. She built dormitories, she built churches, she built hospitals. And she was *hepped* on birth control – and so, inevitably, Mrs Sanger got in touch with her early in the 1950s.'

Actually it was the other way round. Mrs McCormick got in touch with Margaret Sanger, from Boston, in October 1950. They were, in any case, already acquainted: Mrs Sanger had grateful memories, she said in the course of the correspondence, of Mrs McCormick's 'wonderful generosity' in the early days of the birth control movement, 'when we struggled so for the prestige and names like your own'.

Mrs McCormick's purpose in 1950 was to ask Margaret Sanger's opinion on 'two questions that are very much with me these days'. They were: 'A) Where *you* think the greatest need of financial support is today for the National Birth Control Movement; and B) What the present prospects are for further birth control research, and by research I mean contraceptive research.'

Margaret Sanger's reply sped promptly back from her house in Tucson, Arizona: 'I consider that the world and almost our civilization for the next twenty-five years, is going to depend upon a simple, cheap, safe contraceptive to be used in poverty-stricken slums, jungles and among the most ignorant people.' Warming to her subject, Mrs Sanger swept on: 'I believe that now, immediately there should be national sterilization for certain dysgenic types of our population who are being encouraged to breed and would die out were the government not feeding them.'

As for who could do with money for research: well, she would start with $25,000 divided among five or six university laboratories, 'definitely to be applied for contraceptive control'. The laboratories would be 'in this country, in England or in Germany' – the latter an unexpected choice so soon after the war, though a cynic might suspect that Mrs Sanger had in mind that country's ill-gotten experience of sterilizing undesirables.

Luckily, no scheme for mass sterilization, or compulsory (and permanent) contraception ever got off the ground. But soon afterwards, Mrs McCormick was taken to meet Pincus. As we have seen, according to Mrs Pincus, the two ladies told her husband they wanted quick results: but science, he explained, did not work that way. Repeatedly Mrs McCormick demanded to know how much it would cost to set a new line of research going. Repeatedly Pincus avoided giving an answer. At length, goes Mrs Pincus's version of the incident, '"Right off the cuff," he said, "and off the top of my head, $125,000." She brought out a cheque book and wrote a cheque for $40,000 and said, "This is the end of the fiscal year, I will talk to my financial man and you will get the rest." And he did.'

At any rate, Pincus began in earnest to work out a new approach to fertility control. For this he enlisted the aid of Dr Min-Chueh Chang. Recruited from Cambridge University in 1945, Chang intended to stay just for a year in Shrewsbury, but he is at the Foundation still, a tall, polite, smiling Chinese intellectual who after nearly twenty-five years' experience of the American dream still looks a man apart. He has acquired a random assortment of the Western world's accoutrements – a pipe, a black beret, a Rover car – and manages them uneasily like unfamiliar stage-props, while his hold over spoken English is a little precarious.

Pincus lured Chang from Cambridge with the promise of a fellowship at Clark University. It sounded grander to Chang and his student friends in England than it really was. He had arrived from China, alone and with no knowledge of English, at the beginning of the war. But he had the gift of being able to handle, with extreme precision and finesse, small and delicate preparations of animal tissue. At Cambridge he had been studying artificial insemination and sperm capacitation; on arrival at the one-year-old Worcester Foundation he was handed a carbon copy of the research project Pincus had him down for. It was perfusing cow's ovaries to make them release eggs, finding the eggs, mixing them with sperm, fertilizing them, then transferring the fertilized ova to different cows. 'Very imaginative! Very far-reaching!' Chang exclaims with what could be irony, but one can never be sure. 'This was one year's work. I thought it was my whole life!'

However, the project was being run for a rich Texan: Pincus wanted quick results. After several months' hard work at the bench, Chang and two of the other Worcester biologists had managed to induce ovulation in one cow ovary. He wrote later, 'Dr Pincus was pleased and everyone was excited and happy', adding in a characteristically ambiguous comment, 'except me perhaps, because I did not try to find the egg.'

Chang's heart was not in the perfusion project and he asked Pincus to release him from it. To do what? Pincus wanted to know. To continue his study of the fertilizing capacity of sperm. Pincus replied with a joke. Did Chang know what his old Professor in Germany had said to him after a year's work in his laboratory? He had told Pincus he was very fertilizing. While Chang worked this out, Pincus stroked his moustache and studied Chang's outline of the proposed new experiments, which included fertilization of rabbit eggs as a way of examining the behaviour of sperm. Having read it, he told Chang he would find him some rabbits to work with, but he could do the research in his spare time. Meantime, carry on perfusing the cow's ovaries. But, Chang argued, before experimenting on large animals you should try out the experiment on small ones. Pincus gave in: 'Okay, do it your way and have fun.'

Fun was probably not quite the word. For all Chang's patience and skill, with cells of microscopic size, results were slow to emerge. Chang laboured on, seeing little of Pincus. But when he wrote what became a celebrated paper on the effects of seminal plasma and rabbit serum on the fertilizing capacity of rabbit sperm, he asked Pincus to add his name. Pincus said no, it wasn't his work, adding the rather startling explanation, 'You are a sperm man and I am an egg man.' For a time few special assignments came Chang's way and he began to feel forgotten. One day, however, Pincus walked into his room with Margaret Sanger and Mrs McCormick, who told Chang he must be having lots of fun. That word again! Not a man to be patronized, and having already won himself a reputation for his work on reproduction in mammals, Chang said icily he hoped the work would be useful nevertheless.

It was not long before the research to which Pincus had so reluctantly agreed did begin to pay dividends. Fired by Margaret Sanger's warnings about the approaching catastrophe, Pincus drew up with Chang what he described as 'a modest project proposal' which was put to the Planned Parenthood Federation. Mrs McCormick's money had not yet materialized. So, with the initial aid of money from the PPF, work on chemical contraception got under way.

Whoever deserves the credit for the original idea, the actual laboratory work which was to culminate in the pill was done by Chang, who placed it carefully on the record that the first experiment he did was on 25 April 1951, adding (in a note on his association with Pincus published a few months after Pincus's death) a quotation from Confucius: 'Do not get upset when people do not recognize you.' Again the inscrutable comment was added: 'I hope Chairman Mao will say the same.'

Probably it was Pincus's suggestion that the starting-point should be the paper published in 1937 by Makepeace, Weinstein and Friedman, of Pennsylvania, demonstrating that progesterone, if injected into rabbits, would stop them ovulating even though they had been mated. Oestrogen, the other female sex hormone, would prevent ovulation – as we have seen, this was known from experience of treating women with dysmenorrhoea – but there were risks, not the least of which was a possible, if remote, link between oestrogen and certain types of cancer. But progesterone was another matter, and Pincus considered that the Pennsylvania experiment had been unjustly ignored. Chang repeated it, and established new facts about the dose of natural progesterone needed to inhibit ovulation and about the timing of the dose. If it were given by mouth, between two and five thousandths of a gramme were needed per rabbit. (In fact the hormone is more active by mouth in rabbits than in humans.) But if it were injected or deposited in the rabbits' vaginas, it had to be given at least five hours before they copulated and in a dose of between one- and two-thousandths of a gramme. This dose could be given up to twenty-four hours before mating and still work. And the bigger the dose, the longer the period of effectiveness. It was also possible to establish that a pellet of progesterone lodged under a rabbit's skin would inhibit ovulation for a matter of months.

The research paper carrying this information was published

in 1953. The data, Chang supplied. The paper itself was con-
structed (his own word) by Pincus. But the work did not stop
there. From rabbits Chang moved on to rats. Unlike rabbits, the
females do not have to copulate to produce an egg: they are
'spontaneous ovulators', and therefore biologically a step
nearer human beings. Chang's female rats were caged up with
males – two males to every five or six females. Some were given
progesterone and some were 'control' animals, who were given
dummy injections. Once more, injected progesterone stopped
the animals from ovulating, and for periods proportionate to
the dose they were given. By mouth, progesterone was still
effective, but a bigger dose was needed.

While all this was going on, a few miles away in Boston a
physician at the Free Hospital for Women was at work on what
at first sight looked like an entirely different problem, the use
of hormones to correct infertility in women. The physician was
Dr John Rock, Professor of Gynaecology at Harvard and in
charge of the Free Hospital's infertility clinic, a dignified, am-
bassadorial figure and a Roman Catholic.

Rock had come to the conclusion that some otherwise inexplicable cases of childlessness were due to under-development
of the womb and the Fallopian tubes, along which the egg
passes after ovulation, the site of fertilization in healthy
women. Normally, it was known, the start of pregnancy was
signalled by a surge in the production of the female sex hormones, progesterone and oestrogen. As well as this, the uterus
and the Fallopian tubes increased in size. So, if progesterone and
oestrogen were given to these childless women, Rock argued,
it might possibly bring about a state of pseudo-pregnancy, stimulating the growth of womb and tubes, correcting their dys-
function and making fertilization a possibility.

When Rock tried out this notion, it worked. Not always, but
certainly in enough cases to suggest that he was working on the
right lines. Thirteen out of eighty infertile women who had
been given a three-month course of the hormones and then had
discontinued the treatment duly became, to their delight, pregnant. During the treatment they had indeed gone through the
period of pseudo-pregnancy Rock had expected, with everything

from morning sickness and tender breasts to missed menstrual periods. Thus they had lived three months in a state of chronic uncertainty: the mental strain on the women, not to mention their husbands, Rock considered a serious disadvantage, even though the experiment had satisfactorily demonstrated the 'rebound' phenomenon he was hoping for. What was more, large doses of progesterone had had to be used. Because it was comparatively ineffectual when taken by mouth, doses of three to four hundred milligrammes had to be taken daily.

So the treatment still left a lot to be desired. And at this point Rock, by chance, met Pincus at a local scientific conference. Each listened to what the other had been doing. Rock recited his experiences with the rebound phenomenon. Pincus countered with an explanation of the studies of progesterone. Out of their conversation came the idea that instead of using both oestrogen and progesterone, Rock should try using progesterone by itself. In any case, oestrogen was not without a certain risk, and there seemed good reason to believe that progesterone might work as well as both hormones together to produce the rebound effect in women, as it was doing in experimental animals. Moreover, Pincus suggested, the women should not take the progesterone every day. Instead, they should take it for twenty days, then stop to allow normal menstruation to occur, and not begin again with the progesterone until the fifth day of the next cycle. This would avoid the worry of missed periods, and not knowing whether the 'pregnant feeling' was genuine, or merely the result of the drug.

So the trial got under way. The results of this experiment had something for both Pincus and Rock. As a test of a possible contraceptive substance it must have looked distinctly unpromising, since all the thirty women chosen to take part were barren anyway, and had been for at least two years. However, a month's careful observation of each woman in the Reproductive Study Centre of the Free Hospital showed that at least they were all regular ovulators. But during the trial, ovulation was suppressed in a significant number. To find out whether ovulation had happened or not, numerous tests were performed: the women's basal body temperatures were taken, tiny sections of the endometrium, or lining of the womb, were cut out and examined, vaginal smears were taken and the composition of the vaginal fluid inspected. The tests even included in some cases laparotomy – opening the abdomen by surgical operation – to inspect the women's ovaries. In fact, these investigations gave variable and at times conflicting results: some suggesting that the women had ovulated, others that they had not, though the longer the treatment was given, the stronger the evidence that ovulation had been prevented. Furthermore, not all the women stayed the course. Of those who did, none, not surprisingly, became pregnant while the treatment lasted. But all of them, once the progesterone was stopped, promptly ovulated again. And shortly afterwards four of them did become pregnant.

From Rock's point of view the experiment had proved highly satisfactory. From Pincus's, it was less so. For one thing, about one in five of the women began to bleed before the end of their monthly cycles. Also, it had still been necessary for the women to swallow massive daily quantities of progesterone: the dose was still 300 milligrammes. And worst of all, as an ovulation-preventer the progesterone was far from one hundred per cent efficient.

Then the pharmaceutical chemists came to the team's rescue. Pincus wrote to a number of firms in the hormone business. The question was whether any of the companies had anything to offer which might be an efficient substitute for progesterone. In a short time he had at his disposal no fewer than fifteen progestational compounds, which Chang proceeded to test out on animals. Twelve of them were soon ruled out when they proved less active than progesterone itself. Three were left: Syntex's norethisterone; Searle's norethynodrel; and another Searle product, norethandrolone; a close relative of the other two, but though more active than progesterone, it had nothing like the potency of either of the other synthetic compounds. (Some time later it was marketed by Searle as an anabolic or body-building drug, useful for patients who had become underweight and found it difficult to gain weight again.)

Norethisterone and norethynodrel were put through several more tests on rabbits and rats – and then, on women. After a month's observation to see that they were ovulating normally, four were given each compound. None of them ovulated, though they were given only a fraction of the progesterone dose: forty milligrammes of Syntex's norethisterone and only twenty of Searle's norethynodrel. The same regime was used as with the progesterone: a tablet a day from the fifth to the twenty-fifth day after the start of bleeding.

In October 1955 the International Planned Parenthood Federation (Margaret Sanger's brainchild) was holding its fifth conference. It was to be in Tokyo. Pincus decided it would be good to go there and present the results collected so far, and tried to persuade Rock to come too. Pincus was not altogether sure of his ground. 'He was a little scary,' Rock recalls, 'he was not a physician and knew very little about the endometrium though he knew a great deal about ovulation.' Rock would not go, and advised Pincus against presenting oral progesterone, in whatever form, as a contraceptive. Nevertheless, it seemed too good an opportunity to miss: Pincus went, and Chang went with him. (Mrs McCormick footed the bill.)

From a practical point of view, medical research at this stage had little to offer the individual woman who wanted her parenthood planned. In contraception nothing new had been invented for years, except sophisticated variations of the chemical pessary, to be inserted in the woman's vagina before intercourse. If used on their own these chemicals made a precarious form of protection, and at best they were no more than an extra safety precaution, to be used with the time-honoured 'mechanical' devices, the diaphragm and the condom.

As the 150 delegates and observers at Tokyo listened to accounts from all over the world of the growing population pressure and the problems of getting acceptance for such contraceptive means as they could offer, any despondency on their part could have been excused. Nor was there much cause for reassurance, apparently, when the time came on the penultimate day to hear about what was going on in the research laboratories. Dr (now Sir) Alan S. Parkes, then at the National Institute for Medical Research in London, reviewed research into biological methods of birth control, and ended by saying they offered 'little or no hope of early development towards practical application'. In theory, he admitted, a long-acting, safe compound, which would not have the same risks as oestrogen but would prevent the pituitary gland hormones reaching their target in the ovaries, should cause a condition of infertility and would make a satisfactory birth control pill. 'I need hardly say,' he added, 'that no such substance is yet known'.

Curiously, Chang's contribution – a review of the mechanisms by which fertility in mammals might be controlled – was hardly more hopeful. Our understanding of mammalian fertilization, he told the audience in Tokyo's Masonic Building, was most elementary. 'Unless and until we know more about the basic mechanism of fertilization, or reproductive physiology, and external as well as internal factors that control it, to devise an effective measure for its control is only a hit or miss affair.' There was, however, a passing reference in his report to the possibility of using hormones to control reproduction. Any drug or hormone that could cause the neck of the womb to constrict and keep the sperm out would be a good approach, and there was also the chance of being able to 'blockade' the fertilized egg in the Fallopian tube by using oestrogen (an experiment Pincus had made as long ago as 1935).

And so when Pincus's turn came that afternoon, his paper might have been expected to electrify the meeting. It did not. Emphasizing that it was essentially a report of work in progress from a large group of scientists whose spokesman he was, Pincus gave details of the experiments with progesterone on animals, then human beings. Then he passed on to the synthetic steroids, listed the substances he had tested, gave the results of animal experiments and, finally, reported on the effects of norethisterone and norethynodrel when given to women. On the basis of the doses used, he said, these substances would appear to be more potent than progesterone by a factor of at least ten to fifteen. 'Much more investigation is, of course, needed,' Pincus said, 'but they are thus far the most promising agents.' He finished with a confident conclusion: 'We cannot on the basis of our observations thus far,' he said, 'designate the ideal anti-fertility agent, nor the ideal mode of administration. But a foundation has been laid for the useful exploitation of the problem on an objective basis.'

He went on : 'The delicately balanced sequential processes involved in normal mammalian reproduction are clearly attackable. Our objective is to disrupt them in such a way that no physiological cost to the organism is involved. That objective will undoubtedly be attained by careful scientific investigation.'

But Pincus's optimism was not exactly shared by the *rapporteur* for the session, Sir Solly Zuckerman, then Professor of Anatomy at Birmingham University, and now Lord Zuckerman. 'Promising though they may have appeared at first sight,' he said, summing up the afternoon's papers, 'I think it is . . . fair to conclude that the observations reported by Dr Pincus do not bring us as close as we should like to the goal of our researches.' Everyone could agree that progesterone would inhibit ovulation in rabbits, and even in rats. But women – that was another thing. The tests mainly used by Rock to check whether the women had ovulated (changes in temperature, the appearance of endometrial cells and smears taken from the vagina) were agreed by other authorities to be far from one hundred per cent certain. Neither direct examination of the ovaries in the operating theatre nor measurement of substances passed in the urine, which had also formed part of the test procedure, were much help either, Sir Solly observed. Not until there were very many more results could anyone draw conclusions about the effectiveness of oral progesterone. The same applied to the admittedly promising but less comprehensive results achieved with norethynodrel and norethisterone.

In retrospect the Tokyo meeting seems something of a landmark, in that it was the first public announcement of the work that was to culminate in the contraceptive pill. But at the time few could have predicted the outcome of Pincus's small series of tests. To Sir Solly, the meeting was 'not immensely stimulating' and his chief recollection of the occasion is of 'enthusiastic people who sang in buses'. He explains: 'They had one or two of these organized trips away from Tokyo, going off in a bus. I'm not a good one at buses. Or lots of company. Very few scientists. Or were there lots of scientists? I forget. I think there were a lot of earnest planners of parenthood as well.'

On Pincus's paper, Sir Solly made this comment: 'Well,' he said, 'there was nothing particularly marvellous scientifically about his paper, nor was there anything particularly marvellous about what he was saying. The fact that you could suppress an ovary by means of oestrogen or progesterone – well, you could do it with almost any steroid hormone – that had been known for years and years. Indeed, I'd published the first paper showing you could suppress the primate ovary in the thirties. One knew then one could use progesterone or oestrogen or androgen. I used all three to study their effects on the monkey ovary. What was new was the mode of administration.'

At the time, Sir Solly took the opportunity to sound what could have been interpreted, in the light of subsequent events, as an ominous warning. 'We need better evidence,' he told the Tokyo meeting, 'about the occurrence of side-effects in human beings. It is not enough, so it would seem to me, that we take presumed negative evidence about the lack of side-effects from animal experiments to imply that no undesirable side-effects would occur in human beings. There is an urgent need for prolonged observation before we draw any firm conclusions.'

It is ironical that the same cautions are being uttered fifteen years later. But still, said Sir Solly, in a not exactly felicitous phrase, the various reports showed they were no longer groping in the dark: there were definite and promising leads to go on.

That was certainly Gregory Pincus's opinion as he went back to Shrewsbury, not the least depressed, to more trials with the synthetic oral progesterone on which he and Rock had made, as he thought, such an encouraging start.

# 3. Goody's Daring Enterprise

'*We recognized right from the start this was going to be as contro-versial as hell, and we moved very cautiously. If anyone had told us the pill was going to be discussed at bridge parties and across dinner tables, well, frankly, we would have disbelieved it*' –

G. D. Searle Company spokesman, 1969

'*Make haste to use your new remedies, before they lose the power of working miracles*' –

19th-century physician

'When Pincus started,' says Dr Howard J. Ringold, a research chemist formerly at the Worcester Foundation and now head of Syntex's Institute of Hormone Biology, 'if you had asked ninety-nine people out of a hundred whether an oral contra-ceptive was feasible, and acceptable, the answer would have been "No". Pincus had the vision to see that the idea would work. And he had the drive to see it was carried out. Of course after it was all over, there were people who said, "I showed ovulation-inhibition was possible in the rat", and so on. But say-ing the accomplishment is possible is not the same as having the foresight and the imagination to actually do it.'

Pincus died in 1967 of an obscure disease of the white blood cells called myeloid metaplasia, having, by Dr Celso-Ramon Garcia's account, worked himself too hard ('He thought he was indestructible,' Garcia says). Since then, his reputation has un-dergone something of an eclipse. When *The Times* printed his obituary on 24 August that year it referred to 'The Pincus Pill'. Not many would call it that now, save for a faithful band of personal friends and co-workers, and his widow, who feels badly about the inroads into her husband's achievement. 'The lies that went on, and still go on!' Mrs Pincus complained, in a room full of Pincus's books, photographs and mementoes of

their journeys abroad. 'The people that take credit for work
they did not do! He used to say, "Take it easy, baby, it can't
hurt me, you do not understand the human ego, it is irrepres-
sible." But – it's going on still. And he can't get up from his
grave and say what really happened.'

Among the workers at the Worcester Foundation Pincus
could inspire an almost reverential respect. 'He was kind, generous, tolerant, understanding, driving, dedicated,' said one of his
personal staff wistfully, while Anne Merrill, the laboratory
technician who collaborated in most of the early trials with the
pill and its precursors, said to me, 'I pity the people that
haven't known him, really I do.'

He has been referred to as the kind of scientist who is at his
best as an orchestrator of other people's ideas. But this does not
quite do justice to Pincus's part in the work at Shrewsbury in
the nineteen-fifties. Carl Djerassi sums him up as 'a scientific
entrepreneur in the best sense', a man who deserves the credit
for pushing on vigorously with what might otherwise have remained just an intriguing idea. Retrospectively he could be accused of having pushed on too fast. In any event, by the time
Pincus returned home from Tokyo in October 1955 he was
not only optimistic but determined to lose no time with the investigations into the contraceptive use of synthetic steroids.

What he and Rock now needed, as the reception of the Tokyo
paper had made pointedly clear, was more human subjects on
whom to try the progestogens. Between them, Pincus and Rock
collected a group of some sixty women. These consisted partly
of medical students; but they also included a group of patients
probably best described as 'volunteers', from a mental institution near Worcester. Permission was obtained from relatives to
perform on these women what was still by any criterion an
experiment. Whether the choice would now be ethically
acceptable is a matter of opinion.

There were seven women mental patients in this trial. Their
ages ranged from eighteen to forty-three, and all were classified
as psychotics, suffering from some serious chronic mental disorder such as manic depression or schizophrenia. None of them
was having intercourse and assessment of the pill's effects was

limited to such things as measuring the length of their menstrual cycles and changes in temperature, taking biopsies of the uterus and analysing various substances passed in their urine. The pill had the by now expected effect of suppressing ovulation and none of the women seemed any the worse for the test.

Not content with this, Pincus also selected sixteen psychotic men from the same mental institution as the first male 'guinea-pigs' for the pill. Eight of the sixteen received dummy tablets and the other eight were given 10 milligrammes of norethynodrel a day. Some of the latter group were later switched to dummy tablets during a trial which lasted in all for five and a half months. With these, Pincus recorded a definite sterilizing effect as a result of swallowing the daily pill. One young man who went on taking it for the whole five and a half months was found at the end to have smaller testicles than when he started. His scrotum had become 'soft and babyish' in texture and his prostate – the gland which supplies part of the seminal fluid as a vehicle for sperm – had atrophied. As experimental subjects, the psychotic men were not very satisfactory. It proved impossible to get a specimen of their semen, so that the number of sperm could be counted and hence their potency estimated. The psychiatrists at the hospital kept an eye on the men and recorded how often they masturbated. This told them nothing, because the men masturbated as seldom, or as often, on the pill as off. One forty-one-year-old who, again, had been given the full twenty-two week course, was reported by a nurse to have behaved in 'a very feminine fashion'. The others showed no obvious changes in behaviour. The psychiatrists reported no change in the patients' mental state: they were just as psychotic after five and a half months as they were when the trial began. Altogether, it can hardly be reckoned the most informative trial in the pill's history, but it may rank as the most peculiar.

Small groups of patients like these, and especially with these disadvantages, were not the answer to Pincus's problem. Much more substantial results were necessary if the Worcester group were to convince the scientific community that they were really making progress. While tests went on with the women in and around Boston, Pincus looked around for somewhere which would do for the more extensive field trials. The choice fell on Puerto Rico.

Numerous reasons have been given for this. Pincus and Rock wanted to test the steroid regimen on poor and uneducated women. It was all very well to tell the sophisticated Bostonians to take the pills once a day for a fixed number of days each month, then start again after a prescribed interval. The problem was whether this would work when the consumers were feckless and illiterate, and would not necessarily understand the method or remember to take the pills regularly. The ideal contraceptive, after all, would have to suit millions of women in the deprived countries where the population problem was at its worst. Also, the trial should be carried out in a place where the population was reasonably static, but where the birth-rate was high and the women most likely to be interested in a new form of contraceptive. Puerto Rico was one of the most densely populated countries in the world. All the requirements appeared to be met.

But whichever place was chosen, the women were going to be asked, whether they knew it or not, to take part in a gamble. Little was known about side-effects. The tests carried out up to this point had been of short duration. No woman had taken the synthetic steroids for longer than a few months. Whatever the exact form it took, the final product would be a year-in, year-out medication and one could only guess at the long-term effects of suppressing ovulation more or less indefinitely. And whatever the region selected it was essential to keep a careful watch over the women taking the pills, so that the doctors would have as much warning as possible of any adverse effects.

It is not beyond credibility that an area meeting all these requirements could have been found among the white, English-speaking majority of Americans. But Puerto Rico it was, crowded, impoverished and ripe for an intensive birth control programme – a prototype underdeveloped country on America's own doorstep.

The researchers themselves say they had no qualms over the decision. Rock has written: 'I had worked with progesterone and testosterone for so many years before I obtained enough of the former in tablets large enough to be useful by mouth, that I had no hesitancy whatever in using it. Before I went to Puerto Rico we had also done enough with the contraceptive preparations containing the newer progestins to give us confidence that there would be no adverse effects.'

There was another reason for choosing Puerto Rico, which carried weight with some of the team, though not, by all accounts, with Pincus himself. At the time when he and Rock flew down to San Juan, the capital, doctors who spoke publicly about birth control still 'spoke out' about it and often felt it necessary to give warning that their views, and indeed the whole subject, might be unpalatable. 'This is an indignant book!' is the opening sentence of one popular work on contraception, published in 1959 by Dr Alan F. Guttmacher, now chief of Planned Parenthood-World Population, then head of a large gynaecology department. 'It is high time that men of goodwill burst the medical, political and religious shackles which bind them, to analyse and solve health problems by frank, free and unbigoted discussion,' he declared hopefully. 'Perhaps my book will advance that day.' In the mid-fifties birth control was the kind of subject which in many places could not be discussed without a good excuse. Ironically, in this respect the most conservative of states was Massachusetts, where Pincus and his associates had already lit a time-bomb under the tea-tables of those who believed contraception to be a form of self-abuse. More obstinately than any other state, its legislature clung to the beliefs of the Comstock era, surviving in a state law which threatened five years' jail, or two and a half in a house of correction, or fines up to $1,000, for anyone foolhardy enough to purvey contraceptive articles, which were bracketed with implements or drugs for abortion. As usual, the worse-off suffered and money could be used to bend the law. In Massachusetts, as well as Connecticut, where similar laws remained on the statutes, 'people able to afford the care of a private physician', Guttmacher noted in his book, 'can have their needs illegally satisfied in hundreds of doctors' offices, but the poor and the uninformed find themselves unable to obtain what hospitals and community birth control clinics would otherwise be able to provide'. It was a safe bet, he added, that some of the lawmakers who opposed 'the democratization of contraceptive advice' were themselves the eager recipients of illegal birth control information on the quiet. Not until August 1966 was the Massachusetts law amended, in a move which Planned Parenthood acclaimed as 'sweeping the board clean of the nation's last remaining serious statutory restriction on prescription of birth control'. Even then, under the amended rules, advice could only be given legally to married persons. Anyone who extended it to the unmarried still risked, in theory at least, incarceration or fine. Only one other state, Wisconsin, retained this restriction.

With the rearguard of Comstockery still fitfully in action, contraceptive research had to be not too obvious: a large-scale trial of a new 'easy' contraceptive could hardly have been feasible in Massachusetts itself, and Puerto Rico had the extra advantage of being safely out of sight of the bluenose brigade.

Pincus and Rock accordingly got in touch with contacts of theirs in San Juan, where there was a university with its own medical school. Both men flew down there, the project was explained, approval given and help promised. The person appointed to supervise the trial was Dr Edris Rice-Wray, a woman doctor who held a university appointment but was also medical director of the Puerto Rico Family Planning Association and director of the Public Health Field Training Centre. Dr Rice-Wray, one of those fiercely committed women who have ever rallied round the banner of birth control, had been given *carte blanche* to set up whatever family planning programmes she thought practical.

Also assigned to take part was the young physician-gynaecologist at San Juan, Dr Celso-Ramon Garcia. In the form originally arranged, his assignment lasted only two weeks, for Garcia almost immediately wrote to Rock in Boston asking if he could go and work there. Rock agreed and Garcia became one of the key members of the group.

The four of them – Pincus, Rock, Garcia and Chang – made a varied quartet, encompassing clinical and laboratory research, with Pincus as the grand strategist. Looking back on it all a few years later, Chang wrote of Pincus: 'Without his wide knowledge of endocrinology, his organizational ability, and his good relations with the pharmaceutical industry as well as the medical profession, and above all, without his daring enterprise, all this work would be on the library shelves.'

The four men also had the scientific standing and personal contacts required to manage a difficult feat of public relations. 'The studies created an aura of, shall I say, displeasure,' Garcia said to me. 'People had to be convinced that work on contraceptives was not a form of immorality.' In the circumstances Rock's courtly persuasiveness and Pincus's sloe-eyed charm were invaluable assets. It was also a remarkably harmonious collaboration: rows were few and the alliance between the four of them seems to have been bathed in a quite genuine mutual respect. The doubts and anxieties were private ones. Rock, a Catholic, had to convince himself that he was not doing anything intrinsically immoral. Chang was uneasy that the work was a way of putting money into the pockets of the pharmaceutical industry, though (as Garcia tells it), 'Pincus pointed out that this was for the good of society and was a necessary evil.' Chang has never fully accepted the argument: the present-day oral contraceptive regimen of twenty-one pills a month, he says with his reproachful smile, makes business for the drug houses and some more economical method badly needs to be found – 'but then,' he adds apologetically, 'I am a black sheep'.

No doubts of this kind got in the way of Pincus, Rock and Garcia as arrangements for the Puerto Rico trials moved on, with the laboratory work now left behind. This time, however, there would be not two compounds on trial, but one: norethynodrel, the product submitted by G. D. Searle and Company, with whom Pincus now had a close connection. Syntex's entry, norethisterone, was dropped. The reason given was that in animal tests it was believed to have caused enlargement of the testicles in male rats. It was suspected that the compound might therefore have mildly masculinizing effects, and although this has never proved significant, it was enough to tip the scales in favour of the Searle product, despite the fact that both were equally powerful as progestational agents. Any drug which might have tended to produce masculine characteristics in the women taking it, such as deepening of the voice, or growth of hair on the face, obviously would not do. Moreover, Pincus was biology consultant to Searle, not Syntex.

Then a curious discovery was made. It appeared that during the production of the progestogen, a tiny amount – fewer than two parts in a hundred – of oestrogen had intruded. When it was discovered, production methods were revised and the contaminant removed. But now, surprisingly, the pure steroid did not work so well on its own. Women who took it began to notice irregular or 'breakthrough' bleeding, and it even seemed doubtful whether ovulation was still being suppressed. Oestrogen was known to suppress ovulation: the obvious answer seemed to be to put the oestrogen back, but in a controlled quantity. In fact, as later events in the first British trials were to show, controlling the oestrogen was easier said than done, but it was an ironical situation. Progesterone in the first place had been intended to replace oestrogen. Now it appeared that the idea had not worked after all. And when the oestrogen was put back, the effect was that at the end of a twenty-four-day cycle of pill-taking the women, with a few exceptions, bled normally – much to their relief, for the bleeding reassured them that they were having regular periods and were not pregnant, and that everything was as usual.

Whether everything was as usual is a nice point. The withdrawal of the synthetic hormones after twenty-four days mimicked the situation at the end of the monthly cycle when the concentration of natural hormones in the body falls to a low level and causes menstrual bleeding. The difference now was, of course, that the hormones were being introduced from outside. It was a kind of pharmacological conjuring trick. But with a rather important proviso: conjurors know how their tricks work.

It was not clear in 1956, nor is it clear now, precisely how the pill has its effect. The assumption was that in some way, introducing synthetic hormones from outside deceives the body into not producing hormones of its own. There may also be an effect

on the mucus in the cervical canal which diminishes the
sperms' ability to fertilize the egg. But in 1956 the trick was
assumed to be working by a mechanism which smothered the
pituitary gland's subtle control over hormone output.

The natural system hinges on a delicate balance of hormones
secreted in turn in the pituitary and the ovary. First a hormone
is produced in the pituitary, the gland at the base of the brain,
which triggers off activity in the ovary. In the ovary, oestrogen
is secreted. When the amount of oestrogen in circulation
reaches a certain level, several things happen. By a reciprocal,
or feed-back, mechanism, the pituitary ceases to produce the
original hormone and then produces another which shortly
afterwards, at about the middle of the menstrual cycle, causes
a follicle in the ovary to release an egg. The follicle then turns
into the corpus luteum, a gland capable of producing progesterone, which is needed to prepare the womb for a fertilized
ovum.

So it was thought that to give these hormones in synthetic
form throughout the cycle would jam the feedback mechanism.
It was as though the pituitary were being continuously hood-
winked into thinking the appropriate levels had been reached.
Not only reached, but surpassed. The quantity of synthetic
hormones circulating when a woman is on the pill is similar to
the amount in circulation later in pregnancy, when they are
both plentiful and constant. Hence, pill contraception is described as a condition of pseudo-pregnancy, an explanation
which, according to one of his former colleagues at Worcester,
Pincus preferred, disliking and indeed brushing aside the
slightly disturbing idea that a delicate system of physiological
balance had been put to sleep.

Either way, a number of questions are still up in the air and,
in the tactful phrase of medical leader-writers, not yet completely understood. Still less were they understood in 1956 when
the Puerto Rico trials began, using Searle's norethynodrel with
1.5 per cent mestranol as the oestrogenic component, the whole
compound patented as 'Enovid'.

The precise location of the trial was Rio Piedras, a suburb of

San Juan where a large slum-clearance operation was under way, involving an ambitious new housing project. Here, Dr Edris Rice-Wray considered, the women would be easily accessible and unlikely to move. The original object was to collect one hundred patients, but for various reasons the women who were enrolled kept dropping out. And so new names were continually being added.

Luckily, the superintendent of the housing project was enthusiastic about the contraceptive trial. Dr Rice-Wray and her team were supplied with records of the families in the new flats and every help was promised from the staff. All the women chosen to take part were under forty and many of them had been getting conventional, barrier-type contraceptives from the family planning clinic. Each had had at least two children. All of them were given a complete physical examination to make sure they were in good health.

Few of them had ever had such an examination before and they arrived for it dressed in their best and pathetically grateful for the attention. Among the women were some sad cases, sad but typical of San Juan's overburdened mothers. One, Herminia A., was thirty-two and had five children, three of them by a previous husband. She did not want any more because her second husband had been three times admitted to a mental hospital. Another, Julia G. though only thirty, had ten children, aged from sixteen to ten months. 'The husband,' says the casenote, 'is very ill, drinks heavily and makes life difficult for the wife.' Mrs G. had to do odd jobs to support the family, and although she and her husband had daily intercourse he would not allow her to use any form of contraception. Only after a great deal of persuasion was he made to agree to her taking the new tablets.

The doling out of 'Enovid' started in April 1956. Each woman had a month's supply of twenty 10-milligramme pills with instructions to start taking one a day five days after the first sign of monthly bleeding, and then stop at the end of the month. Not everyone understood completely: one woman thought she only had to take the pills when her husband was home – he travelled frequently, she explained: 'I didn't take them when he was away. I took them when he was here, of course.' She became pregnant.

The women were warned they might experience various side-effects. They were told they might feel sick or dizzy and that they might also have stomach pains or diarrhoea. The warnings seemed to make little difference to their willingness to take part, though there were some dropouts. Out of 109 women who stopped taking the pill, twenty-five did so because of the uncomfortable effects they had been warned about – although another thirteen women who also had the side-effects stayed with the trial and found the reactions less and less troublesome as the months went on. Nine husbands disapproved and in six cases the woman's own doctor advised her to stay out of the trial. In three cases, the woman's priest told her to have nothing to do with the whole sinful business.

As was bound to happen, news of the trial reached the ears of a local journalist. When he telephoned the Secretary of Health to check the story he was surprised to find, as well he might have been, that the Secretary, a Dr Pons, knew nothing about it, and was annoyed that public health nurses were being used on the project. Pons promptly telephoned Dr Rice-Wray, who agreed that the trial was in progress and that she was directing it. But, she told him sharply, she was doing so in her own time, apart from her public health duties. When Pons protested that it was difficult to see how the two could be separated, he was told that they were living in a democracy and any government employee had the right to use his spare time as he liked.

Pons was quoted next day as saying that he did not think it proper for government staff to engage in ' neo-Malthusian' activities, nor did he approve of the Health Department being 'used as bait' for such a project. Several patients withdrew from the trial. Shortly afterwards, incidentally, Dr Rice-Wray took up an appointment in Mexico, a WHO post as Medical Officer for the Dominican Republic, Haiti, Cuba and Mexico itself.

Meantime, however, more and more women began to ask for the pill, and Dr Rice-Wray and her staff started a waiting list of those eager to take part. Dr Rice-Wray reported later: 'Sometimes people say to the patients, "How do you know what this is? It might be dangerous." This does not bother most of those who can reply, "I have been taking it eight or nine months and I am happy and I don't get pregnant."'

Among the doctors and technicians managing the trial, realization began to grow that this was more than a scientific experiment: it held the possibility of profound social change. Anne Merrill, the Worcester Foundation laboratory worker who was one of the group which flew regularly to San Juan, told me: 'I would see these young women with many, many children, although I wouldn't know they were young women until I'd looked at their records. Some of them looked like what I would think of as a great-grandmotherly type, you know. All wizened up and gaunt to the point where you wanted to do something for them. I'd think it was due to old age, but then I'd look at the records and the woman would be thirty-four, you know, with ten children.'

As the months went by the observers began to see a change in the Puerto Rico wives. Anne Merrill said:

'To see these women after they'd been on for a year ... You know, to get them through one year, without having a baby! And the fact that they themselves realized they'd gone this whole year and they weren't pregnant, and here they were, hale and hearty! But the exciting thing was that, for instance, some lost their babies in a flood, and they decided they wanted another baby and they just stopped the pills. And then we started seeing the babies that were arriving, and they'd be fine.

'I can remember the first time we worked out statistics and found out that we got fifty-fifty proportion of boys and girls. Because there was this terror – are you going to get all girls, or all boys, you know, what's going to happen?'

These unguarded recollections underline how much of an experiment the Puerto Rico trial was. Nobody quite knew what would happen to the women and guesswork played a surprisingly large part in the proceedings. Even the dosage used has been described by one of the team as 'a shot in the dark': 10 milligrammes of norethynodrel plus 0.15 milligrammes of the oestrogen, mestranol. Lower doses were tried soon after the first field-trial was complete. First 5-milligramme, then 25-milligramme 'Enovid' was used, and since then there has been a steady trend towards lower dosage. (By 1969, the FDA recorded in its Second Report on Oral Contraceptives, more than ninety per cent of the combination tablets being prescribed contained 2.5 milligrammes, or less, of the progestogen. One of the most recently approved products contains one-third the dose of oestrogen and about one-tenth the progestogen in the original pill.)

In Puerto Rico, to the delight of all concerned, the contraceptive effectiveness of the new pill was clearly demonstrated. Reviewing what had taken place, in January 1957, the doctors had before them the records of altogether 221 women who had taken the pill for periods up to nine months. Dr Rice-Wray's conclusion was this: 'Adding the number of months of those patients who have been taking "Enovid" more than two months, we have a total of forty-seven patient-years. During this time we have not had one single pregnancy that could be attributed to method failure.' There were seventeen pregnancies due to 'patient failure' – women who had stopped taking the pill and promptly become pregnant.

Dr Rice-Wray summed up: '"Enovid" gives one hundred per cent protection against pregnancy in 10-milligramme doses taken for twenty days of each month.' But she added a cautious rider: 'However, it causes too many side-reactions to be acceptable generally.'

It may seem an unexpectedly pessimistic conclusion, but it was true that just over seventeen per cent of the women who had taken part up to then had had unpleasant reactions of one kind or another – thirty-eight women out of 221. Many had had more than one reaction. Twenty-nine had felt dizzy, twenty-six had felt sick, eighteen had had headaches and seventeen had actually vomited. Nine had had stomach pains, seven had felt weak and one had had diarrhoea. This added up to a far from negligible burden of minor illness, but the women had all been told they might expect to feel symptoms of this kind: therefore, it was possible that many of those who complained of reactions were exhibiting a 'placebo effect'. They would have felt the same, perhaps, if they had been given placebo (or dummy) tablets and warned to expect to feel off-colour.

At all events, the trial was not only continued, but extended. More women were accepted and another trial was set going in a small town called Humacao a few miles south east of San Juan, under the direction of a certain Dr Adeline Pendleton Satterthwaite. As this proceeded, a plan was concocted to test the 'placebo effect'.

By this time, Dr Rice-Wray had left for Mexico. In her place Dr Manuel Paniagua was now Director of the Family Planning Association. With Pincus he devised a scheme by which one group of women who were using conventional contraceptives were told they were to be given 'Enovid' as well. The idea, Dr Paniagua told the women, was to find out if they were suited to this kind of tablet. Meantime they were to carry on using the contraceptives they normally used, just in case 'Enovid' would not do for them. The usual warning about possible side-effects was given. However, the pill they were given was not 'Enovid' at all, it was a dummy pill made of lactose. But seventeen per cent of the women duly reported unpleasant reactions.

Another group were then given genuine tablets, but this time, no warning of side-effects was given. And the actual incidence of those effects was a little over six per cent.

Watching the progress of events in San Juan with more interest than most was a group of men in Chicago: the top marketing and public relations executives at G. D. Searle's headquarters. The growing success of Pincus's Puerto Rico trials confronted them with what seemed in turn an agonizing dilemma – and a breathtaking opportunity. It did not need much business acumen to see that, potentially, this was one of the biggest things that had ever happened to the pharmaceutical industry: God's gift to whichever firm laid hands on it first.

What they had in their laps was one of the classic golden eggs of the drug business, something in the great, money-spinning tradition of aspirin, penicillin or purple hearts, but with advantages none of those possessed. If the idea could be sold, the pill would have a virtually guaranteed sale to millions of women at the rate of 240 tablets a year throughout their child-bearing lives, from menarche to menopause, with only such intervals as a woman chose in order to have a baby. And the pill was something more: a drug to be taken, for perfectly valid reasons, not by the sick, but by the healthy.

But there was a large question-mark: would it be acceptable? Birth control was still, the businessmen reasoned, a delicate subject. The word contraceptive suggested rubber goods from a back-street shop, not a tablet from a leading pharmaceutical company. Searle's public relations expert James W. Irwin says: 'We were a company with an absolutely impeccable reputation. G. D. Searle and Company had built its name as a speciality house. We had the information from the Puerto Rico trials as authority and we relied on Pincus's opinion as to the medical end. But the policy decision had to be made right here in this office. We were going into absolutely unexplored ground in terms of public opinion.

'So, to be quite honest, we played it by ear. We underestimated the receptivity of the product. We got quite a surprise.'

'Enovid' was placed before the US Food and Drug Administration with an application for its licence as a contraceptive product. It had already, since 1957, been licensed for use in treating menstrual disorders and a good deal of evidence had been collected of its effectiveness in conditions such as threatened abortion and dysmenorrhoea. Backing up the new application was an account of the experimental work and the Puerto Rico trials.

In 1960 the FDA gave the drug its approval for contraceptive purposes. Its use was to be limited, the FDA ruled, to two years for any one person, a ruling that was not relaxed for some years. Searle executives were already paving the way for a careful marketing campaign. A series of symposia had been held at the Chicago offices where results of trials with 'Enovid' had been pooled and discussed. Much of the emphasis had been on the gynaecological uses of the product. But the real point was the contraceptive effect. Then, as the launching date for the product grew nearer, James W. Irwin went to work on the public relations.

'My fear was that this would provoke an avalanche of letters to the editor,' he says. 'So, I went to see various people. I sat down with a lot of my friends at the *Saturday Evening Post*: they did two major pieces about the pill. And I said, "Look, I want to warn you, this is controversial, you may get a sizeable protest." And there was none.

'I told the same thing to *Reader's Digest*. And there was none.

'We were overly cautious. All my experience told me that you could not do this without getting your teeth knocked out – or some of them. And we didn't lose any teeth.'

The misjudgement was understandable. Searle had failed to appreciate several factors. One was that the impression had got round that the pill was the new, modern contraceptive that did not get in the way of sexual pleasure. Wives who were on it began to rediscover sex, not only because they no longer had any worries about becoming pregnant, but also because it was all so easy. It was not like using a contraceptive at all in the usual sense. There were no barriers, nothing to be inserted or put on, there was no fiddling about beforehand with chemicals or caps, no precautions had to be taken – except to swallow the pill as directed. With one blow, it seemed, the scientists and doctors and drug manufacturers had made sex into what ordinary people thought it always should have been – a source of sheer pleasure, not a biological necessity invented to maintain the species.

Furthermore, Comstockery really was at its last gasp. Contraception may have been, as Searle's executives warily pointed out, technically a forbidden subject in Massachusetts, Wisconsin, Philadelphia and the Dakotas. But the veils were being lifted and attitudes to contraception and sex in general were relaxing. The arrival of the pill was not an isolated event and one did not have to look far for the first signs of the permissiveness of the sixties. (As the Searle company were laying their plans for marketing 'Enovid', Penguin Books in London were making equally careful plans for marketing that year their 3s 6d unexpurgated edition of *Lady Chatterley's Lover*.) The change was already gathering momentum as the sixties began, brought about by far more complex influences than the invention of the contraceptive pill. Nevertheless G. D. Searle and

Company stepped in at exactly the opportune moment. Today, they can afford to be complacent. 'I'm pretty sure that when history books are written,' said their chairman John G. Searle a short time ago, 'our organization's greatest single contribution to mankind will be "Enovid". It is a positive answer to a world threatened by overpopulation, and the resulting poor subsistence, poor shelter, and poor education that surplus peoples are forced to endure.'

Syntex, the only other drug company seriously in the field at the time, were shouldered aside. They had done the original development work and if it had not been for the efforts of a succession of Syntex chemists, from Russell Marker onwards, there would have been no Puerto Rico trials. Unfair on Syntex perhaps, but unlike G. D. Searle and Company they were not ready for the moment when it came. 'Through the mid-fifties we were busy fools,' said one of their executives ruefully, 'selling vast quantities of raw materials for other people to make a profit out of.' They were not a retailing company, they had no marketing organization, no 'detailmen' to visit doctors and push the company's products and no large-scale advertising or public relations set-up. Searle, on the other hand, had been in business since the eighteen-eighties, when an Indiana pharmacist, one Gideon Daniel Searle, had founded the organization and done well selling medicines in the form of tablets and lozenges rather than fluids and powders.

In any case, as even their rivals concede, Searle took a gamble with the pill. If the gamble came off, they deserved the jackpot. Syntex executives privately express their professional appreciation of Searle's courage in taking the first step. Their own efforts to interest the dignified and long-established firm of Parke, Davis and Company in a joint agreement to market a pill based on norethisterone came to nothing. Parke, Davis thought the hazards too great. And in the negotiating process Syntex lost a valuable two years. Not until they concluded a licence deal with Ortho Pharmaceuticals, a company already selling contraceptive jellies and creams, were they ready to take a share of the business they had in a sense created. Meantime Searle had the advantage, and they played it for all it was worth: 'Enovid' *was* the pill, *they* were the inventors. From virtual stagnation their share prices went up with a rush and reached a new peak by 1964, a year in which their net profits were well over $24 million, a figure exceeded more than once in the next four years.

Well before this, other trials of 'Enovid' had started, one of them in Port-au-Prince, Haiti, where 'Papa Doc' Duvalier was persuaded that a birth control programme would make sound economic sense, at the same time affording an opportunity to score off the Catholic Church, with which he had broken a few years earlier. An approach was made to Pincus and his collaborators, a committee of Haitian officials was appointed and a trial of the pill set going. Unhappily, although it made a promising start, this did not last. The Boston team became alarmed when they discovered that the medical system was under political control: for instance, death certificates could be signed by all kinds of unqualified people ('almost any politician could sign,' says Garcia, aghast) and still more alarmed by the tendency of people involved in the trial to disappear suddenly, including the chief administrator, a former chief of the Haitian Air Force. In 1969 only one member of the original committee of four survived and the records of the project were in a state of irretrievable confusion.

Elsewhere other clinical investigations were less at the mercy of political caprice. In Los Angeles, encouraged by the preliminary reports from Pincus's group, Dr Edward Tyler started a trial with norethisterone and norethynodrel, along with three other, newer progestogens with somewhat weaker effects. Tyler's Family Planning Centre in Los Angeles was already a well-established proving ground for contraceptive methods, although since the work had been started in the early nineteen-fifties there had been very little to test except specially prepared vaginal creams, jellies and foams. Tyler, a merry individual and at one time a professional gag-writer who furnished jokes for Groucho Marx, says he was 'easy prey for anyone who approached us with a reasonable contraceptive idea that merited investigation'. The pill certainly did. But his initial experiences with it were not terribly promising. By June 1958 he was reporting to the annual meeting of the American Medical Association on 715 women, all relatively fertile, about three-quarters of whom had been given 'Enovid' or 'Norlutin' (now the trade name for norethisterone), as contraceptive compounds. But 474 of the women did not continue with the drugs, and the biggest single group of these, 177 in number, stopped taking them because of various side-effects, mainly nausea and diarrhoea or irregular bleeding. Another fifty women gave up because of 'loss of confidence in it, caused by neighbourhood gossip, hearsay tales of difficulties encountered, and reports in papers and periodicals emphasizing the experimental nature of the pills' – although, Tyler pointed out, the patients had all been told the drugs were experimental before they started.

What was more, twenty-two of the 241 women who stayed the course became pregnant. But nothing loth, Tyler went on with more trials and by 1961 was ready to report, with seven other doctors, on 570 women who had been taking 'Norlutin' for various periods up to four years. The grand total represented altogether 7,194 'patient-cycles'. Many of the women were long-term users and now, Tyler's impression was that the side-effects – this time, nausea, weight-gain and menstrual irregularities – made little difference to the pill's usefulness. The side-effects were relatively uncommon (only 1.1 per cent for nausea, and eight per cent for the menstrual troubles). Also, he noted that these effects had no serious consequences. Tyler and the other doctors had gone out of their way to ask some of the women if they had had unwanted effects: this may have exaggerated their importance, he admitted, 'but we thought it desirable to err in that direction'.

But the most noteworthy thing about Tyler's report was the extremely low failure rate. Out of the 570 women, only six became pregnant without intending to. This worked out, to use the formula adopted by contraception specialists, at a failure-rate of 1.1 per hundred woman-years.

In Puerto Rico and Haiti, Pincus had by this time collected statistics covering 25,421 monthly cycles. With these, the failure-rate was 1.7 per hundred woman-years. Dr Rice-Wray, who had launched a trial in Mexico City, reported a failure-rate of 0.6.

These figures were remarkable enough when compared with the failure-rates of conventional contraceptive methods. (In Puerto Rico a 1961 study had given failure-rates of 33·6 per hundred woman-years with the diaphragm, 42·3 for vaginal suppositories, 36.1 for vaginal creams and jellies and for the humble condom or french letter, 28·3. Better results were usually collected in more sophisticated places, but the 1961 Puerto Rico figures only served to sharpen the comparison with the results using the pill.) What made the new results even better was the well-founded suspicion that pregnancies were nearly always due to the patient's oversight, not a failure of the pill. If the women took their pills regularly and conscientiously, the failure-rate was generally nil.

Needless to say, the pill was big news. And the more it was talked about, the greater was the demand. By the end of 1961, it was estimated, 408,000 women in the USA were taking oral contraceptives, and by the end of 1962, 1,187,000 – a number which had almost doubled within another twelve months. By 1965 Dr Sheldon J. Segal, Director of the Population Council's Bio-Medical Division, computed that American women were consuming progestogen and oestrogen tablets at the rate of 2,600 tons yearly. One of every four married women under the age of forty-five had used or was using an oral contraceptive and the actual users at that time numbered some 3·8 million. 'American women,' he concluded, deadpan, 'are interested in oral contraception.'

In Britain, doctors prominent in the family planning move-ment had followed the initial series of trials with what one of them described as 'interest and caution'. And as early as 1959 the Council for the Investigation of Fertility Control had decided that it was safe to embark on carefully controlled clini-cal trials in Britain. By now, total experience of 'Enovid' in-cluded over 20,000 cycles in which it had been administered to over 1,000 women. Of these women 150 had had the pill for twelve to twenty-one consecutive cycles and sixty-six had had it for twenty-four to thirty-eight cycles, or over three years.

The first British trial of any size took place in Birmingham under Family Planning Association-CIFC auspices and was directed by a group of doctors from Birmingham University headed by Dr Peter Eckstein. Searle paid, and supplied the pills.

The project was to contain a few surprises. When it started, forty-eight women were involved, all under thirty-six, all with at least one child and all in good health. To qualify for inclusion they were also required to live within easy reach of Birmingham and, of course, as doctors politely put it, to be exposed to the risk of pregnancy. To be precise, they were expected to be having sexual intercourse at least once a week. One woman amazed the doctors by logging on her specially provided record card that she had intercourse during the trial ninety-one times in one month, a figure considered so extraordinary that it was left out of the final calculation in case it ruined the figures for average frequency of copulation (about once every fourth day). The doctors decided that this woman's unusually full sex-life had nothing to do with the pill. 'It must surely have had something to do with the husband's libido,' thoughtfully observed the then Medical Secretary of CIFC, Dr Eleanor Mears.

The tablets given to the Birmingham women were 'Enovid'. They contained 2.5 milligrammes of progestogen and 0.05 milligrammes of oestrogen. At least that was the intention. But something went wrong with the manufacturing process. It turned out that the tablets contained only 0.036 milligrammes of the oestrogen. Within a few weeks, fourteen of the women were expecting babies.

In some alarm the organizers summoned all the women to the clinic and broke the news to them. They were advised to finish the current cycle on the pills they already had, then the thirty-four who had escaped pregnancy (not unexpectedly, this group did not include the woman who had so upset the averages) were switched to pills which contained 5 milligrammes of norethynodrel and 0.075 milligrammes of mestranol. None of these became pregnant.

However, the results demonstrated that, in these women at least, norethynodrel with inadequate oestrogen would not prevent pregnancy. There was a growing body of opinion based on findings in Puerto Rico with a lower strength tablet, that the oestrogen content could safely be cut; and some intriguing questions were raised by these events about possible differences in susceptibility between women of different ethnic types. But the fate of the fourteen Birmingham women who now, no doubt with mixed feelings, embarked on pregnancies they had not expected, showed that the magnitude of the oestrogen component of the pill was critical. From other effects noted during the trial it seemed that the compound used had not suppressed ovulation but only delayed it. (It later appeared that norethisterone, unlike norethynodrel, probably did remain an efficient contraceptive when it was given with insufficient oestrogen to suppress ovulation completely.)

The real irony of this discovery, once again, was that it was the oestrogen which apparently was having the main contraceptive effect, the ingredient which was supposed to be supplanted by the progestogen and had originally got into the pill by mistake. Yet the accident in Birmingham did supply an opportunity to study the course of thirteen pregnancies which had occurred after the mothers had been on a prescribed course of the pill. (One of the pregnant fourteen was believed to have failed to take the tablets regularly.) Three of the pregnancies miscarried, a figure which excited no comment from the six doctors who reported the results in the *British Medical Journal*. The other eleven mothers produced twelve babies between them; one had twins. All the babies were well after apparently normal pregnancies, and the proportion of boys to girls was exactly fifty-fifty.

As to the general acceptability of the pill among British women, the trial was highly encouraging. There were side-effects: the commonest was headache, often but not always accompanied by a sick feeling and complaints of swollen and tender breasts. Some women also had backache and cramp-like pains in the abdomen, and there were also complaints of dizziness and vaginal discharge. But the doctors noted that as the trial went on the symptoms tended to disappear.

Also, the women as a whole, many of whom had joined the trial because they were not happy with conventional contraceptives, liked the pill. 'Throughout the trial,' wrote the doctors, 'they continued to express their preference for the tablets, in spite of experiencing various and occasionally disagreeable side-effects.' More remarkable still, they remained enthusiastic even after it had become clear that the pill, at least in the strength they had been given, was not always infallible. 'Several stated spontaneously,' went the report, 'that they felt "well" or better than they had before beginning to take the tablets.'

Addressing the Society for the Study of Fertility in June 1961, Dr Eleanor Mears went further. 'Many patients,' she said, 'have expressed themselves as being absolutely delighted with the freedom from contraceptive measures related to coital acts, of being more confident and relaxed at intercourse, and other interesting observations have been made – for example, discharge gone, skin improved, hair less greasy, abdominal post-operative pain gone, feeling better than ever before, first orgasm ever, cut down smoking, dysmenorrhoea gone.' The real test was whether the women persevered with the pill, she added: and 'So far, the results are encouraging.'

Encouraging indeed. So much so that by the time the report of the Birmingham trial appeared in print, the Family Planning Association's Medical Advisory Council had recommended that the pill should be offered as a method of birth control in FPA clinics. The recommendation covered 'Enovid' – to be called 'Conovid' in Britain – and other similar combinations of progestogen and oestrogen. Closely studied research, said the FPA, should go on to evaluate the effects of long-term consumption of the pill, and it was to be given under strict medical supervision, they insisted. Only 'suitable cases' should be given it, and then by 'medical staff trained in the method'. There was also a caution that the pill should not be given unless the clinic was well enough organized to deal with the 'administrative problems'. In other words, there had to be the staff and the facilities for keeping a check on the women taking the pill, besides giving them the complete medical examination implied in the phrase 'suitable cases'.

However, hedged round with cautions though it was, the pill

had now arrived in Britain. There was no official body at this time for approving new drugs. Though America had the FDA, Britain did not yet have the Committee on Safety of Drugs, which was set up as a result of the thalidomide disaster. (It was at the time when the pill was approved by the Family Planning Association that reports of the unexpected effects of thalidomide were beginning to circulate.) Not until January 1964 did the Drug Safety Committee go to work. In the meantime, the FPA's sanction of the pill had the effect of official approval.

Searle released a series of medical journal advertisements and mailing shots to British doctors, advertising the pill in a 5-milligramme dose of norethynodrel with 0.075 milligrammes ('a very small quantity', the leaflets stressed) of mestranol. 'Conovid', said their leaflets, this 'achievement of Searle research' was 'the responsible answer to a universal problem'. Hand in hand below the slogan, a young couple walked confidently away towards the future, their happiness assured by 'the most effective contraceptive known to man'.

In the jargon of the drug industry, the pill was an 'ethical specialty', meaning it was advertised to doctors only and sold on prescription, not to the general public. Therefore it could not be advertised directly to the customers, but in view of the huge publicity the pill had already had, this was a trifling disadvantage. Thousands of women who had been impatiently waiting for the chance to try it went to their family planning clinics or family doctors to ask for a prescription. The question of acceptability that had so worried the manufacturers seemed laughably irrelevant.

# 4. An Awful Lot of Acorns

*'As for the pill, while we know some of its short-term side-effects who will presume to say that we have reaped the full harvest of its late sequelae?'* –
British Medical Journal, June 1968

*'From the point of view of the health of society it would be more justifiable to have oral contraceptives in slot machines and restrict the sale of cigarettes to a medical prescription'* –

Dr Malcolm Potts, October 1968

By the time 'Conovid' was launched in Britain, enough statistical information had been accumulated for the makers to claim confidently that its effectiveness as a contraceptive was beyond dispute. 'Studies over the last six years involving 30,000 cycles of experience,' said a Searle handout, 'have shown that "The Pill" provides a degree of contraception never previously achieved.'

Averaged-out figures showed that the pill was far superior to existing methods of contraception. Searle's publicity material cited figures using the statistically exact but bewildering formula of 'failure-rate per 100 woman-years': the number of accidental pregnancies times 1,200 (100x12), all divided by the total months of exposure. Translated into simple terms, the figures could be interpreted thus: in twenty-five years of marriage, a woman using the 'rhythm' method to plan her family would have, on average, six unplanned pregnancies. A couple practising coitus interruptus, historically Europe's most popular contraceptive technique, could expect between four and five. If the husband used a condom, three or four.

But with the pill, the failure-rate was so small as to be negligible.

Effectiveness even approaching that of 'Conovid', Searle

proudly claimed, 'has never been reported for any other method of contraception'. Moreover, all the other methods available, whether mechanical or chemical, 'have demanded for maximum reliability a skill and care that many have found either inconvenient or unreliable'.

But was the pill safe? The makers were confident on that score. 'There has been no evidence,' the leaflets declared, 'of dangerous long-term side-effects with "Conovid".' Trials had shown, said Searle, that there was no impairment of subsequent fertility: women who decided they wanted to have a baby could stop taking the pill and they would be as fertile as ever. Pregnancies after taking the pill had been normal and the children born had been healthy.

But nobody really knew what the future held in this respect, just as nobody could say with any certainty exactly how the pill was working ('a brief period of pseudo-pregnancy appears to be induced', was Searle's explanation). The point was that it did work: women who took it regularly and according to instructions, it was continuously reiterated, did not become pregnant. In any case, the ingredients were only synthetic versions of substances already present in the human body. Science, you might say, was merely imitating nature.

And yet, and yet . . . There were still many questions left, and in leaving them up in the air, indeed by bringing out the pill at all, medicine had got itself into a giant dilemma. Once it was out, a product so useful and so attractive, appealing to such deeply-seated human motives, was going to be used. But nobody would know if it was safe to take for, say, twenty years until twenty years had gone by, with many thousands of women taking it, and so the safety question began to go round in circles. One could only wait and see.

People began to talk nervously of 'the biggest experiment in mass medication in scientific history'. Few other medicaments were like this: there were perhaps a few roughly similar precedents, such as the chlorination of public water supplies and, just about arguably, mass immunization against infectious diseases. Even so the pill wasn't quite the same as either. Admittedly, it too was to be taken by healthy people: they were not ill, just unwilling to be pregnant. But taking the pill, unlike being immunized or drinking disinfected water, was interfering with something fundamental to woman's sexual personality. The complex and finely adjusted balance of hormones was being smothered, and in what some doctors suspected to be a summary and even brutal fashion.

These fears remain. When a London newspaper invited its women readers to send in their doubts and queries about the pill in 1968 an avalanche of letters reached the office which the woman journalist assigned to the story summed up as follows: 'You swallow the pill and you *know* you are not going to have another baby. Your skin glows and now you can love your husband with warmth and spontaneity. Then the doubts begin ... is it right what you are doing ... can you go on for years and years "interfering with Nature", as your mother calls it. You push those strange symptoms you are feeling out of your mind. Next month you will see the doctor again and – well – you might be run over by a bus tomorrow anyway. Risks are part of life. So you concentrate on thinking of the happiness the pill has given you. This, basically, is the story hundreds of women have told me in the letters about the contraceptive pill.'

The pill had been available for public consumption only a matter of months before doctors realized that the emotional state of the women taking it was a major factor in the effect it had. Dr Paniagua's artful experiment with the placebo pills in Puerto Rico, when he showed that women who expected side-effects duly experienced them whether they took the pill or a placebo, was the first of a number of similar investigations. In Mexico an experiment was launched in which some 1,700 women were given dummy tablets, thinking they were the pill. Between twelve and fifteen per cent of them reported back to the doctors that they were having breakthrough bleeding.

Not only can the woman's own attitude make a difference to the side-effects she experiences: the way the doctor talks about the pill can be just as powerful an influence. One woman doctor told me: 'There is one of my colleagues who can be persuaded to prescribe the pill – if the woman is persistent and makes enough of a nuisance of herself. But as she hands the prescription over she says, "Go on then, but mind you, I *certainly* wouldn't take it myself." Well, it doesn't surprise *me* that her patients get headaches galore, nausea, depression, the lot.'

A striking example of the opposite point of view can be found in Dr Caroline Deys, a Cambridge doctor who has run family planning clinics and who is married to the Medical Secretary of the International Planned Parenthood Federation, Dr Malcolm Potts. Dr Deys announced in April 1970 (when the fortunes of the pill seemed to be on the slide again) that she had been giving oral contraceptives to her two-year-old daughter for about a year. She had done it to prove to other women that the pills were harmless and the child had had ten or twelve of them altogether. 'I know exactly what is in the pill and I know exactly what it does to women,' claimed Dr Deys. 'It should not cause any harm. I think most children during their lives take aspirin and other things which are much more dangerous than giving her an odd birth pill.'

Inevitably too, the press gets the blame for spreading 'alarming' stories about the hazards of taking the pill. 'Every time some fool of a journalist writes something knocking the pill, I groan,' said a doctor in a family planning clinic. 'I know perfectly well I can expect a sad little stream of patients next day wanting to know if they're going to die of heart failure or cancer, go bald or have a stroke or something. There are far too many alarmist and irresponsible reports about the pill's side-effects.' The drug houses, too, feel hard done by in this respect. 'The pill,' grumbled a public relations man in Britain, 'has been without question the most shot-at drug in history. It is amazing how the papers seize upon critical letters and declarations and boom them up, yet to a large extent they ignore the favourable news.'

One of the medical staff of a pill firm, also in Britain, was equally piqued by what she regarded as 'biased' reporting. It only took one case where a woman's death from a blood-clot in the lungs was attributed to the pill, she complained, 'and the press goes mad, plastering the coroner's comments all over the paper. But an article in one of the medical journals, based on a good, reputable series of patients which gives the pill a clean bill of health – that's just not reported.'

For quite a time incidents in coroners' courts have been a cause of despondency and irritation among the pill's manufacturers and its other supporters. Headlines like 'Pill Caused Woman's Death – Coroner', appearing on average three or four times a year, have caused much wincing in boardrooms and do no service to the carefully wrought image of the pill as a natural, safe, 'physiological' contraceptive. It was mainly to combat the cumulative effect of this kind of thing that in February 1968 the pill manufacturers took action: with a certain amount of mutual wariness they sat down around the same table to form the Oral Contraception Information Centre, dedicated to providing 'a reliable source of scientific data and balanced objective information on oral contraception for all communications media'. But the idea of providing information, when asked, on every aspect of the pill – even its dangers – was not unanimously welcomed by the five participating companies, who, remarked the public relations man in charge, 'saw us in the role of a fire brigade putting out coroners' fires'.

That was a desperate hope in any event. The disturbing headlines kept being printed. At Leeds coroner's court in July 1969, a verdict of death by misadventure was recorded on a thirty-four-year-old mother of four, whose death from a blood-clotting episode was judged by the coroner to have been connected with the contraceptive pill she had been taking. The literature made it clear, said the local family planning clinic doctor, that there were two cases in 100,000 'where one has felt that taking the oral contraceptive has been the cause of thrombosis' – at which the bereaved husband shouted across the court, 'My wife may be a statistic to you. You have killed not one, you have killed five in one fell swoop.' Then he broke down and wept.

Rather surprisingly, the American pill manufacturers have not attempted any collective public relations effort comparable to what has been done in Britain. It has not been for want of trying, according to James W. Irwin of G. D. Searle. 'I would dearly like,' he told me, 'by means of some committee or foundation, to promote through accepted public relations techniques the philosophy of oral contraception. This would take warning of movements contrary to the pill and take steps to alert doctors and so forth, and kind of defuse those movements.' But despite several years of attempting to persuade the pill makers to join forces in a campaign of this nature, the effort has so far failed. Doctors have been left to make up their own minds.

However, taking a decision about when to prescribe the pill is not always easy. If newspaper readers have been bothered by coroner's remarks and reports of medical journal articles, so too have doctors. They have had even more conflicting data to try to sort out than their patients, who do not hear the more or less continuous mutter of comment in the professional weeklies on such arcane matters as the pill's effect on serum iron and total iron-building capacity, on excretion of delta-aminolaevulic acid, activation of carrier proteins and folate metabolism.

Not all of it has any immediate significance (though it might have later on) but the conscientious doctor with several hundred of his women patients on the pill has to do his best to keep up with the minutiae of medical news on the subject and assess the value of it all.

It is probably just as well that the average housewife on the pill sees nothing of all this, unless it is important enough, or peculiar enough, to get into the papers. The sheer diversity of effects reported to be possibly linked with the pill would be enough to scare most women off and send them back thankfully to coitus interruptus, the cap or the condom. This diversity does not surprise the pill's critics. To them it is no more than you should expect from using a powerful synthetic drug, with continuous effects all over the body, to thwart an event – ovulation – which can only happen during a few days in each month.

To such people, the more that is known about the pill, the less trustworthy it seems and the less justified one is in prescribing it. The liver, the kidneys, the circulation, the hair, the skin, the eyes, the breasts, the cervix, the connective tissue, the teeth and numerous other organs or systems of the body have at various times been reported vulnerable to the pill's ingredients, not necessarily to a serious extent and usually in only a small number of women. Not long ago, in response to an inquiry from an eminent research worker, an official of the Drug Safety Committee in Britain listed the reactions to oral contraceptives which had been reported to the committee from 1964 to mid-1968. His list – the type of information doctors like to keep away from patients – is an extraordinary and alarming catalogue of medical conditions. It includes amenorrhoea (absence of menstruation) and other menstrual disorders, breast disorders, weight gain, oedema (excess fluid in the tissues), depression, headache, migraine, unusual skin pigmentation, nausea, thyroid disorders, diabetes, porphyria, anaemia, thrombosis and haemorrhage of the blood vessels in the brain, high blood pressure, clotting of the veins, clotting in the lungs, coronary thrombosis, inflammation of the arteries, jaundice, skin disorders, hair disorders, tumours, abnormality in a baby, abortion – and, last but not least, pregnancy. Inclusion in this list does not mean that any particular condition can necessarily be linked with the pill. But most of them would be recognized by doctors as conditions for which they should be on the alert.

Some of the case-histories from the literature on the pill could well have come from the pages of a volume on the curiosities of medicine. In Copenhagen, two pill-taking sopranos were discovered to be below the level of peak performance – literally, for they were unable to produce their top notes. The theatre's medical adviser was called in and he advised them to stop taking the pill: when they did, the vocal changes were halted within a week.

More remarkable was the patient of a doctor in Milwaukee, who complained that whenever she sat up or turned over in bed, or indeed whenever she sneezed, she could feel, and hear, something crackling in her chest. When she was examined, the doctor found no sign of anything wrong except that part of her breastbone seemed slightly loose, a discovery disquieting enough for him to question her more closely. It emerged that she had been on the pill for eighteen months, and she was told to find some other method of contraception. Was the pill to blame? The doctor did not commit himself : he was waiting to see if the crackling would go. Meantime he pondered the possibility that this curious symptom might be related to the relaxation of the pelvic joints during pregnancy.

In some respects the Milwaukee doctor's experiences paralleled those of a Manchester dentist. One of *his* patients was found to have a condition resembling 'trench mouth', with sore gums and loose teeth. It appeared she had been dosing herself with twelve times the usual daily quantity of norethynodrel (where she had got it was not reported). Chairside experience had frequently shown, the dentist commented, that women who were having their teeth straightened were at an advantage if they were pregnant: the teeth are 'slung' from ligaments in the jaws in rather the same way as the joints of the pelvis, which are loosened during pregnancy. It was as though the guy ropes supporting the teeth had been slackened, he remarked. (A publicity man at G. D. Searle promptly picked up the story and circulated it with the cheerful catch-line Pill May Help To Straighten Teeth.)

One of the most bizarre findings, however, and apparently not so rare, came from the Leeds Regional Blood Transfusion Centre in 1968. The Director of the Centre, Dr Derrick Tovey, wrote to the *Lancet* to report that one in every hundred of the blood donations reaching his laboratory had plasma that, instead of its usual straw colour, was green. Most of the green plasma at Leeds, it turned out, came from women on the pill, who made up around six per cent of the donor population. Statistically this suggested that one in six of women on the pill might unknowingly be in the same condition. Plasma is the portion of the blood, just over half of it, which is *not* red or white corpuscles. It is often given in transfusion and its extraordinarily varied components include proteins, salts and antibodies, as well as waste products and traces of iron, copper and zinc. But why had this particular plasma turned green? It was not entirely clear, except that it seemed possible that the plasma contained less than usual of its yellow pigment, and, perhaps, more than usual of a particular protein which is blue in colour. Maybe this was some idiosyncratic response to the steroids in the pill. Nor were the Leeds blood transfusion experts the only ones to notice this curious phenomenon. A few months later an associate professor of pathology at Stanford University Medical Center in California was reporting a similar discovery. He believed the green plasma was still suitable for transfusion. No one who had been given it had come to any harm so far, he said, when given green plasma units from his blood bank. Nevertheless, whichever way one looks at it, green plasma can hardly be considered normal. Whether it is anything to worry about remains unclear.

As the pill's advocates frequently protest, one must beware of the anecdotal approach. The reports cited here do not necessarily mean that all women on the pill face an equal risk of their voices deepening, their teeth falling out or their blood turning green. Individual case-reports reported in the medical weeklies need not have any significance except to the patient described. In any case, the doctor who reported them may have been mistaken.

In his textbook on contraceptive practice Dr Malcolm Potts, Medical Secretary of the International Planned Parenthood Federation, quotes the case of a doctor who gave a woman a prescription for 'Enovid' and was alarmed to discover six weeks later that she had a thrombosis of the veins. On further investigation it emerged that her pill-prescription had in fact never been dispensed.

Also, for good or ill, the pill makes women notice their symptoms more – symptoms they may have had for years without consciously realizing it, or which may be quite unimportant. 'Some women who are taking oral contraceptives admit that they feel guilty in doing so, and this attitude of mind gives rise to a further group of symptoms – so-called scapegoat symptoms – which are the result of increased self-observation.' Thus the *British Medical Journal* in 1968, commenting this time on the possibility of a link between the pill and bald patches on the scalp: no link has been firmly established and indeed it may even be that taking the pill provides some inexplicable form of protection against this condition. Yet the general impression remains, said the *British Medical Journal*, that the two are connected.

Next to some of the graver side-effects which have been reported, such a symptom as a small bald patch might seem of little account, especially to a male doctor dealing with a tiresome, apprehensive woman patient. The same applies to discolouration of the skin, a relatively common complaint with the pill in certain countries which doctors have been known to dismiss as a mere cosmetic aberration which can easily be concealed. At least it has a medical name to give it more substance: chloasma. In its textbook form it consists of symmetrical blotches which appear mainly on the face. Not infrequently it occurs in pregnancy, and it seems that certain pigment cells react more readily to sunlight in the presence of higher levels than normal of circulating hormones. It is infrequent in Britain, but in countries blessed with more sunlight it is not. One medical journal described it as 'a daily dermatological problem' in Australia, which for its size has the largest pill-taking population in the world.

Occasionally, the discolourations do not go when the woman stops taking oral contraceptives. Women who freckle easily tend to do so more easily still when they are on the pill and the freckling can merge into chloasma. One Australian doctor has helpfully suggested that women who have this problem should not only avoid sunlight but also take their pills when the sun has gone down – so that exposure to the light occurs when the circulating level of hormones is on the wane.

Explanations for the side-effects which are reported in such bewildering variety constantly founder on one basic difficulty: in the present state of medical knowledge it is impossible to be sure exactly what is happening to the steroids in the pill once they get into the body. This is not only because not enough is known about the pill. Not enough is known about the body either.

This applies to medicines other than the oral contraceptives. Developments in molecular biology in the last twenty years have brought within scientists' grasp a much more intimate knowledge of bodily processes than was dreamt of previously. Alas, in the case of drugs and their actions the full fruits of this knowledge have so far proved elusive. In a general way, doctors know that, for example, aspirin relieves headaches by depressing activity in the central nervous system, and brings down a fever by acting on the heat-regulating centres of the brain. But how it acts on those centres or what it does in the central nervous system no one can state dogmatically. The same is true of countless other drugs. To a large extent, medicine is still an empirical science: doctors use a drug because they know it works.

Conversely, doctors do not use a drug either because it does not work or because it can be seen to have too many unwanted effects besides those that are required. The difficulty is to decide when the unwanted effects can be accepted, and when they cannot – to decide when the discomfort or danger of an otherwise useful medicine cancels out its benefits. The decision with the pill is basically the same as with many other drugs. As Dr C-R. Garcia remarks, 'Clinical medicine at this point in time is very much a gamble. The physician is being called upon all the time to make these value judgements. And people are losing sight of the fact that medicine is not an exact science – not yet, though I guess it might come with computers.'

Because of the paucity of rock-solid, provable scientific facts about the pill's effects on minute body processes – which is where the hunt for a cause always ends up, or rather, peters out – statistical surveys have been the backbone of research on the pill. Here the computer *can* take over. Hence, the bulk of the agreed data on the pill consists of studies with series of patients in whom observable effects have been recorded and compared with those in carefully matched 'control' patients; their statistical significance has then been measured according to well-defined if somewhat esoteric rules. But even if medicine is on firmer ground with figures than it is with molecules, there has still been room for dispute.

Exact analysis of the pill's effects has not been made any easier by proliferation in the types of contraceptive pill. Since 1960, when 'Enovid' was approved by the FDA in Washington many more brands and varieties of steroid contraceptive have entered the field. There has been, too, a steady tendency towards reduction of the doses used. The International Planned Parenthood Federation lists in its medical handbook thirty-two varieties of the 'classical' pill combining a progestogen with oestrogen in a single dose. Thirteen progestogens, in doses ranging from one to ten milligrammes, are in current use in these pills, but only two oestrogens, the lowest dose here being one-twentieth of a milligramme and the highest, one milligramme – but the two agents differ in their oestrogenic potency. From 'Aconcept' to 'Zyklo-Farlutal', well over a hundred trade-names, protected by patent, have been coined, aimed at suggesting the product's pharmaceutical role as well as achieving the distinctiveness and memorability preferred by sales managers.

These hundred-odd names cover, in addition to the 'classical' combined pill, thirteen types of what has been a little boastfully called the 'second generation' of oral contraceptives, so-called 'sequential' pills. While the classical pills are taken for twenty to twenty-two days, according to the brand, followed by a six- to eight-day pause, a packet of sequentials contains two kinds, to be taken successively during the same month. The first contains oestrogen alone and has to be taken for the first fourteen to sixteen days. From then until the end of the cycle the woman has to take what is in effect the classical pill. The idea is to mimic more faithfully the output of sex hormones in a normal month, in which oestrogen production is followed by progesterone. Though it sounds admirable, it is not such an effective contraceptive as the original twin-steroid combination and the pregnancy-rate among women on sequential pills is slightly higher – whether because the women have left too long an interval between courses, or because of some intrinsic failure of the method, is not at all clear. Moreover, since it was established by the Committee on Safety of Drugs that high-oestrogen pills carry a higher risk, use of the sequential varieties has fallen out of favour.

A 'third generation' of contraceptive pills exists too. The first of these made its appearance comparatively recently (in 1969) and contained no oestrogen at all. Marketed under the reassuring name 'Normenon' and nicknamed the 'mini-pill', it consisted of a small dose of progestogen (one already used in some sequential pills) and nothing else. The woman was told to take it daily, year in year out, with no break at the time of menstruation. Syntex, makers of 'Normenon', called it 'a "continuous-use" conception regulator'. It did not prevent ovulation, they explained, but what it appeared to do – and the explanation was hedged around with the familiar qualifications – was to thicken the mucus in the womb so that sperms could not get to the egg. Like the sequential pills, the 'mini-pill' had a higher failure-rate than the original product, it was not supplied in British family planning clinics for this reason. Furthermore it was never finally approved by the US Food and Drug Administration, though it had been extensively tested clinically at some thirty centres in America.

The (probably) temporary eclipse of the 'mini-pill' came in January 1970 when Syntex in Palo Alto withdrew it because of adverse effects in dogs. The effects included possible metabolic changes and the development of lumps in the breasts of beagles. Within a few weeks, Syntex in Britain – where the 'mini-pill' had been authorized by the Drug Safety Committee – voluntarily withdrew it from sale, and 70,000 women who were using it had to find another brand of pill, or another method of contraception. This development was a double disappointment to the manufacturers (and to a number of research workers) because, as will appear, the 'mini-pill' appeared to be a significant improvement on the classical varieties with regard to side-effects such as the level of clotting factors in the blood and alterations in blood-sugar levels.

But to complicate matters still further, individual brands of classical contraceptive pill need not have the identical effect on the same woman. Nor do two women necessarily react in the same way to one make of pill. The oestrogenic effect of brand X may be more pronounced than that of brand Y, and Mrs A's endocrine system is certain to be subtly different from Mrs B's. This makes possible an almost infinite variety of effects, and doctors are enjoined in medical handbooks and by drug firms with more than one type of pill in their catalogues to make sure they prescribe the right pill for each patient. Find out, say the instructions, if your patient has a tendency towards acne, greasy skin and hair, fullness in the breasts and fairly light periods with perhaps cramps in the leg or the abdomen. If so, her hormone balance is likely to favour the progestational side and you should prescribe for her a more strongly oestrogenic pill. If on the other hand she tends to have heavy and irregular bleeding, suffers from headaches and puts on weight easily, then she should have a pill relatively strong in progestational effects.

It would be a naïve person who believed that every doctor prescribing the pill took the trouble to go through this kind of assessment. Either through carelessness, ignorance or lack of time, a vast number of them, to judge from comments by other doctors, prescribe according to habit or whim, and are easily moved by the advertisements they receive from drug companies in the form of note-pads, blotting paper and other desk aids. According to a standard medical joke, which one suspects is uncomfortably close to the truth, one doctor who was asked what principles governed his choice when prescribing an oral contraceptive, answered, 'Oh, I don't know old boy, it depends which blotter I happen to be using at the time.' 'Yes, I call them blotting-paper doctors,' said one consultant gynaecologist, 'it's terrifying really, doctors are far too gullible and some of them are quite incredibly slapdash about this sort of thing.' Nor was it only with the pill, she added feelingly: prescriptions for tranquillizers, sedatives and antibiotics were handed around with equal abandon. 'The whole prescribing set-up in this country needs a thorough overhaul if you ask me.'

Until that happens many women will continue to take the first oral contraceptive their doctor thought of, even though it has been argued (by one of Syntex's medical staff) that as many as sixty per cent of all women who take the pill are on the wrong one, and should by rights change to a pill better suited to their particular hormone makeup. Syntex themselves do have a range of tablet-strengths. If this estimate is correct, many of the pill's minor side-effects are being needlessly endured, and could be eliminated by a change to a different brand. As things are, these reactions are a frequent reason for a woman abandoning pill contraception. What the handbooks list as 'minor', 'trivial' or 'annoying' effects may be none of those things to the woman herself, especially if they seem to give substance to the vague feeling that taking the pill is 'against nature'. Nausea, tender breasts, headache and putting on weight, however, tend to be regarded by many doctors as the unimportant small change of oral contraceptive side-effects, producing no more than minor inconvenience – and once, at least, an embarrassing scene at the altar, as described by a Lancashire girl in a letter to a British woman's magazine: 'My husband and I bought our wedding ring three months in advance and I started to take the pill one month later. By the time our wedding came along, my fingers had swollen (unnoticed) so that only after a struggle were we able to fit the ring on during the service. It became so uncomfortable that during the honeymoon I was forced to remove it and we met with some very embarrassing situations.'

A quandary for the newly-weds, maybe, but hardly more. Most of the 'trivial' side-effects of the pill tend to be confined to the first few months of taking it. If the patient perseveres, they stop. Furthermore, whether a woman gets these symptoms or not depends to some extent on her attitude towards taking the pill. Women who put on weight, Pincus considered, may do so because they are no longer worried about becoming pregnant and therefore have better appetites. (G. D. Searle were still repeating this sunny thought in their package leaflets in 1969.) Says Dr John Rock: 'My standard is this. How does the patient respond to her own progesterone and oestrogen. For example a girl who has oedema, spots and so on, well, girls like that must be careful because the pill will do the same thing. And those who respond rather extravagantly to their own hormones in pregnancy will respond to the pill likewise when they take it month by month by month. Take nausea, that icky feeling, it disappears usually during the third month of pregnancy, and it does on the pill. This is why I was so prompt in recognizing the innocuousness of contraceptive steroids.'

Coming as it does from one of the prime movers of the

original research on the pill, Rock's complacency is not hard to understand. Like nearly all the doctors and biologists concerned in the beginnings of the pill, he takes a generally optimistic view of its possible hazards, and becomes impatient at what he regards as carping criticism. 'Child spacing is a very serious matter,' he wrote not long ago, 'I would therefore beg irresponsible or poorly-informed zealots, however well-intentioned, to cease their presumptuous intimidation of conscientious parents, by wishful speculation supported by quotations from unscientific sources, or from long outdated and later corrected statements of a few reputable gynaecologists.'

However, antagonists of the pill are not so easily warned off. It would be easier to take the hint if tender breasts, feeling sick and extra weight were the only side-effects to be reckoned with. But deeper down may lurk bigger and more dangerous fish: cancer, effects on blood circulation, impaired liver function, diabetes, even, possibly, unknown hazards which have not yet come anywhere near the surface.

Because these dangers have so far proved statistically slight, the pill's protagonists insist on the need to put them in the right perspective. Instead of scaring people with what might happen to a score of women out of every thousand on the pill, the apologists say, we have to remember the enormous benefits of oral contraceptives – not only as a means of controlling population but as a source of positive benefit to individual women. Being free from the worry of becoming pregnant, and being able to enjoy sexual intercourse in a spontaneous and unpremeditated way, are benefits every woman who takes the pill has been led to expect. But by way of bonus, she will probably also have her premenstrual tension relieved and her periods will no longer be painful and miserable. If she has acne, that will probably go as well (unless she is one of the unlucky one per cent in whom it gets worse), and the same goes for women who have faint traces of a moustache. On top of all this, her general outlook will improve, and in the words of one enthusiastic woman doctor in Glasgow, she will 'bloom with health', while any sexual difficulties she has will be smoothed out: 'It makes for a happier relationship and a more stable marriage, which leads to a better family atmosphere for the children.' Another doctor, a Northampton general practitioner, claims that women who take the pill pay fewer visits to their doctors for general health complaints. Looking at the clinical records of 184 women in his practice, he found that their average number of surgery visits was just over eight per year. After they began using oral contraceptives, the visits dropped to an average of three. It was impossible not to be greatly impressed, he told a medical symposium in Liverpool, by the effectiveness of the pill and the way it was accepted, and the 'truly remarkable' change for the better in his patients' lives. 'I have frequently found it difficult to identify in my mind,' he declared picturesquely, 'the alert, jolly and bright-eyed woman calling for a repeat prescription of her oral contraceptive with the anxious, sullen-faced drab who had previously entered my surgery and asked in hopeless tones – as an aside from her myriad complaints – for information on this method of birth control.' 'Nearly all doctors in family planning clinics or general practice, and others involved in marital problems agree,' wrote a medical officer of health in the South of England, 'that oral contraceptives have saved many marriages from permanent breakdown.' Another medical writer went further still, suggesting that the pill might prove a kind of social lubricant, oiling the intellectual machinery of commerce and administration: by making wives happier, he claimed, the pill makes husbands more even-tempered, less preoccupied with their domestic problems and more able to take balanced and responsible decisions at the office.

In some women the freedom and relaxation conferred on them by the pill brings out a covert sexuality their husbands may never have suspected (and, as will appear, may not like). Patients report back to family planning clinics with joyful accounts of 'a second honeymoon', or of having had 'a proper orgasm' for the first time in their married lives. How far the pill really does restore flagging libido has been a matter of some speculation, partly because sexual desire is not the easiest thing to measure in scientific terms. The most accurate standard of measurement is how often a person has intercourse, but even this may not be all that reliable and may be a better criterion of the husband's sex-drive. Early reports on the 'Enovid' trials in Puerto Rico conveyed the perplexing conclusion that half the women had intercourse more often when they were on the pill, but that forty per cent had it less often. In the remaining ten per cent there was no change. Later attempts to find out what the pill was doing to women's sexual appetites have had similarly ambiguous results. At an international conference in Prague in the summer of 1968, a Leipzig gynaecologist, Dr Lykke Aresin, told his audience of 250 sexologists the results of interviews with five hundred women aged twenty-five to thirty, all of whom had been on the pill for at least two years. Half of them said it had made no difference to their sex lives. One in five said their sexual drive had diminished – but most of these were said to have been either latently frigid or having marriage problems such as drunken or unfaithful husbands. One-third of Dr Aresin's interviewees, however, said their sex lives had improved. They had intercourse more often and enjoyed it more, said Dr Aresin, mainly for the simple reason that they no longer feared becoming pregnant.

Women like these have been unrestrained in their enthusiasm for the pill. 'I thank with all my heart, the people who have made this possible,' wrote one contented mother of two to a British daily newspaper. To *Time*'s Latin-American edition, a woman wrote: 'To the pill I can accredit harmony, communication, fulfilment, satisfaction, happiness, stability, understanding, acceptance, relaxation, achievement, compatibility, courage, love, peace, and Christ.' With such a cornucopia up on its end, who can wonder if the beneficiaries see no good reason to deprive themselves of its riches. Dr Edris Rice-Wray in Mexico found the popularity of the product almost an embarrassment during her work with the Maternal Health Association. 'We have some women who have been on the pill for eight years,' she declared recently, 'and we can't get them off them – not even to take part in our study of a once-a-month injection.' A similar dilemma confronted a group of research workers in Oakland, California, where the existence of a well-established health scheme supplied a good opportunity for a large-scale prospective study of the pill's effects on over fifteen thousand women of child-bearing age. The problem was to find the controls: not enough women were *not* taking the pill to provide a matched sample of the 'normal' female population.

After all, the most convincing evidence that women like the pill is the fact that so many are taking it – about twenty million, all over the world. As one distinguished endocrine specialist put it, in an unguarded moment, 'This has got aspirin beaten to a frazzle.' 'In spite of adverse publicity, fear of thrombosis, cancer, varicose veins, and long-term side-effects,' ran a report in *World Medicine* in the summer of 1969, 'a clear two-thirds majority of women taking the pill decided to use this form of contraception on their own initiative. Of the remaining third who decided to take the pill on someone else's suggestion, only half were advised to do so by a doctor ... In spite of the disadvantages they feared or experienced, the majority of the women [in a survey at Slough, Bucks.] – especially in the thirty-six to forty age group – were overwhelmingly in favour of the pill for its effectiveness, convenience, the peace of mind it gave them and the improvement in their marital relationships.'

Many women cling to 'the philosophy of oral contraception' with an affection that no amount of pessimistic comment can shake and to bolster their loyalty they have the approval of a majority of doctors. 'Forty million women can't be wrong,' wrote an Indianapolis doctor (whose enthusiasm had temporarily overwhelmed his arithmetic) to an American medical newspaper a little while ago, 'Let's emphasize the good points!'

One of the most persuasive advocates of the pill's good points is the Medical Secretary of the International Planned Parenthood Federation, Dr Malcolm Potts. By marshalling the statistics for deaths from pregnancy, childbirth and abortion, and comparing them with deaths from the pill, he concluded that there was less risk of death from taking the pill than any other method of contraception except sterilization and legal abortion. Every method of contraception which is not one hundred per cent effective exposes a woman to the risks of death associated with pregnancy and childbirth, Potts declares. 'Once a woman has sexual intercourse she faces death whichever way she turns.'

In a speech to the 4th Asian Congress of Obstetrics and Gynaecology in Singapore in 1968, he put it this way: 'If a woman wishes to have normal marital relations and at the same time chooses not to become pregnant, then she is more likely to be alive in one year's time if she uses oral contraceptives than any less effective method of family planning. To put the same conclusion another way, if all the married women in England took oral contraceptives for one year, then the death rate among women of fertile years would be less than it is at present.'

Potts calculated that, balancing the inherent risks (if any) of each method of contraception against the risks of pregnancy after the method failed, there would be, out of one million women using the pill, twenty-seven deaths. Out of a million using condoms, twenty-eight would die, and so would forty-eight out of a million using coitus interruptus, fifty-six using diaphragms, sixty-four the rhythm method – and so on, right up to the top of the table: 225 deaths due to unprotected intercourse and 240 due to criminal abortion. (The IUD is left out of the calculations because the risk of death is not known.)

An attempt to set the pill's risks into perspective was badly needed but it has not proved at all easy to manage. Statistics have their pitfalls. A woman's fertility declines as she grows older, and the risk of unexpected pregnancy – if a contraceptive method fails – declines also. (On the other hand, the inherent risks of pregnancy increase with age.) Nor are failure rates with the various methods constant. For instance, the effectiveness of mechanical methods such as the diaphragm or condom 'improves' when a couple have all the children they want and therefore have stronger incentives to use those methods more carefully. In the January 1970 *British Medical Bulletin* Potts acknowledged these difficulties. And in his article, co-authored by Dr Gerald Swyer, also an ardent supporter of the pill, less simple conclusions were reached. Although the likely deaths from the pill during one year are small in number (twenty-one out of one million women, the two authors conclude, compared with thirty-three for mechanical methods, fifty-six for spermicides, coitus interruptus and the rhythm method), the picture changes dramatically if induced abortion, legally performed, is accepted as a last-resort measure, to remedy the failures of all methods. The figures quoted this time, giving the risks involved through a married life, with two planned pregnancies, give a total death-rate of 888 out of one million with the pill, and it is the highest of all methods – higher even than the 786 deaths to be expected when no precautions are taken, but when abortions are performed if need be.

Abortion, of course, cannot be regarded as a convenient method of family planning, and with repeated abortions the risks are liable to increase. But Potts concludes that there are three rational possibilities open to a couple who plan to have two or three children. They can use the pill, or the IUD. Or they can use the less effective traditional methods, with induced abortion as a 'long-stop'. Or one of them can be sterilized. 'Each possibility has its merits,' says the *Bulletin* article, 'and in a large community it is likely that all three will be used separately and often in sequence.'

This represents a considerable modification of the original argument, and the final impression from all these figures is that they only reveal the near-impossibility of arriving at definite conclusions on a matter so full of subtle individual variations. But there is an important proviso: that in countries where the risks involved in pregnancy and childbirth are much higher than in Western Europe and North America, different standards are called for. In Africa or India, for example, the balance of safety, if not of suitability, shifts in favour of the pill.

And what about the other risks of life in the twentieth century? Remembering these does offer a paradoxical kind of comfort to many women who swallow their daily oral contraceptive with the same suppressed feelings of unease they have when they light up another cigarette (the risks of which are known with some exactitude). Many other human activities have a high death-rate, but are regarded as harmless and raise no public outcry. 'In the USA,' Potts said in his Singapore speech, 'there are over five thousand boating and swimming fatalities every year, and there is ten times the likelihood of a death in the family if father buys an outboard motor boat than if mother takes the pill.' In Britain, about 1,800,000 women take the pill, which makes it statistically probable on present evidence that each year some forty will die as a result. But about six hundred women of child-bearing age meet a violent death on the roads of England and Wales every year and about five hundred die of respiratory cancer, probably caused in most cases by smoking. Deaths from taking the pill are far less numerous than those which occur through aspirin poisoning, accidental electrocution and suicide, though they are comparable, admittedly, to the number of deaths attributed in official statistics to broken ankles, cold weather, or a blow from a falling or protruding object.

It can even be argued that the pill affords some protection against accidental death or injury on the road, or in the home, office or factory. Women whose menstrual cycles are difficult or painful are known to be more accident-prone at these times than normally. If the pill banishes pre-menstrual depression they could have a better chance of escaping accidental death, the commonest cause of fatalities in women of child-bearing age.

And yet, and yet ... In spite of these arguments the doubts remain and the risks of the pill never seem to be forgotten for long. The pill's defenders accuse those on the other side of Grundyish prejudice. 'You don't hear many people protesting about the other extremely powerful drugs we prescribe,' said one doctor, 'which by the way have been investigated far, far less than oral contraceptives. It's only because this is about sex. A lot of people absolutely detest the thought that a lot of other people are getting more fun out of sex than they are – or than they used to. So they keep uttering horrendous warnings about side-effects. But look at the deaths from barbiturate poisoning every year. Why don't they make dramatic public statements about what dangerous things barbiturates are?'

One knows what he means: if it had nothing to do with sex, the pill would generate much less vehemence than it does. But by no means all those who are sceptical about the pill are nursing obscure sexual jealousies. There is a groundswell of

scepticism, and a sense of disquiet frequently colours the pronouncements of individual specialists as well as official bodies.
Reviewing progress in contraception in 1968 a London endocrinologist wrote sadly, 'Oral contraception is not, it is now
realized, the boon and the blessing to man that at first it was
thought to be.' Side-effects seemed inseparable from contraceptive efficiency and there were 'pointers to a good crop in 1969
and 1970. Big oaks from little acorns grow and there are an
awful lot of acorns.' In America, introducing the FDA's second
report on oral contraceptives in August 1969, Dr Louis M. Hellman, chairman of the FDA's Advisory Committee on Obstetrics and Gynaecology, wrote: 'Concern about the immediate
and long range side-effects of the hormonal contraceptives has
increased as scientific investigations have uncovered a host of
diverse biological effects, and as the drugs have become available to increasingly large segments of the world's population.'
With gruelling memories of the thalidomide episode, doctors
have more cause than ever to maintain what has been called
a high index of suspicion towards the drugs in their armoury.
As one medical editorial put it in May 1968, 'One indictment
of the medical profession is its gullibility ... there is much that
we do not know about the pill, and the profession should be
sufficiently adult to say so. Over-enthusiasm has cost us and our
patients dearly in the past.'

Not long after this, on 1 December 1968, more than seventy
physicians, gynaecologists, endocrine specialists, pathologists,
psychiatrists and others with a professional interest in oral contraceptives arrived for a meeting at the Sheraton Hotel in down-
town Boston. Included in their number were fifteen observers from such agencies as the Ford Foundation, the National
Institutes of Health and the Federal Food and Drug Administration.

Everyone at the meeting, which went on for five days, had
some clinical or research interest in the pill, but in the words of
one of the organizers, the conference was 'for honest men
only'. Its purpose was to look as dispassionately as possible at
the evidence relating to the pill's effects on metabolism – the

complex processes which make up the body's daily traffic in liquids, solids and gases.

The idea for the meeting had come originally from the National Institutes of Health, a body roughly equivalent to, but considerably larger than the Medical Research Council in Britain. Three men had organized the Boston meeting: Professor Hilton A. Salhanick, of the Harvard Centre for Population Studies, Professor David M. Kipnis, Professor of Medicine at Washington University, St Louis, and Professor Raymond L. Vande Wiele, Professor of Obstetrics and Gynaecology at Columbia University, New York. For two years they had kept a watch on the broad lines of current research on the pill and the participants were chosen only if their work seemed scientifically unimpeachable and free of bias.

Advocates of the pill, already dismayed by rumours of damaging information being processed at the Sloane-Kettering Institute for Cancer Research on a link between the pill and cancer of the cervix, viewed the Boston meeting with disquiet, as the mustering of opposition against the 'philosophy' of oral contraception. Significantly, a meeting held 'for reassurance' took place in private a few weeks later in Palm Springs. This was organized by Dr Edward Tyler of Los Angeles: attending it were a number of long-standing champions of pill contraception and it was privately described as 'a reply' to the Boston conference.

But if the two incidents resembled the alignment of forces before a battle, this was not the intention of the Boston meeting's main architect, Professor Hilton Salhanick. One of the biggest obstacles to impartial evaluation of the pill, he declares, is the tendency of medical men to take up immovable postures on the subject. 'I am not against the pill, I am against ignorance, and I think people on both sides have been polarized excessively,' he told me.

I don't say no one should take the pill, I think some women should because the alternatives for them are too serious. People who say we must ban the pill now are wrong, but equally wrong are the people who say all these abnormal findings mean nothing.

There are two questions. One: *are* there any abnormal findings in women on the pill? Answer, yes. Two: are they meaningful? Well, you can't answer that straightaway, I think some are and some are not. I want to see the data, to put it where it can be examined. That was the purpose of our meeting.

To take part in what they described as a 'workshop' on oral contraceptives, Salhanick, Kipnis and Vande Wiele had assembled an impressive array of talent from clinical medicine and research. The list of participants included forty-four full, associate or assistant professors; nineteen were of full professorial rank.

Although Salhanick's plea for impartiality, had it been heard by those who met at Palm Springs six weeks later, may have reassured them, the full story of the proceedings at Boston, when at length it came out, can have given no cause for complacency.

The 750-page tome duly published in August 1969 attracted surprisingly little attention, but it is a summing up of most of the medical case against the pill. It sets out the results of more than fifty separate studies of how the contraceptive steroids, and related hormones, might affect biological mechanisms. Salhanick, Kipnis and Vande Wiele explain a little disingenuously that the work presented is for the most part 'straightforward and noncontroversial', by which they appear to mean incontrovertible: 'the most convincing aspect of the reports included in this work', they state, 'is the consistency with which data were replicated in different laboratories.'

Certain conclusions from the fifty-odd research papers are emphasized by the three organizers. Contraceptive steroids are not, and should not be identified as, natural substances. They are unique, synthetic compounds. They have diverse actions on the human body, whether they are given singly or in combination, and regardless of how much is given, how often, and by what route. Their effort cannot be equated with phases of the menstrual cycle, nor of pregnancy nor any state of 'pseudo-pregnancy'. Furthermore, despite some ten years of use, no one has been able to demonstrate what in medical jargon is known as a 'dose-response curve' – in other words, no one can say exactly what is the relationship between a given quantity of contraceptive steroid and the actual contraceptive effect. There are differences in the degree and type of effect between the synthetic steroids and the natural ones, and to say that the pharmacological state induced by the pill is the same as pregnancy is a 'semantic over-simplification' which should be abandoned forthwith.

Many of the metabolic effects of the pill are peculiar to individuals. But others are commonplace and have been noted in laboratories as far apart as Miami, Florida and Paddington, London. There appears to be a consistent pattern: a challenge to the women's 'physiological reserve' in the form of a constant extra load on the machinery, as though a finely engineered Swiss watch were being continuously made to run, say, one per cent faster than it was designed to do. Said Salhanick and his colleagues: 'When ample reserve exists, the effects are less marked; but when the reserve is decreased for any reason, the effects become prominent. It appears worthwhile therefore to examine the reserve status of patients' systems prior to prescribing such medications and to plan re-examination at measured intervals thereafter.'

The accumulated data suggest that no tissue in the body and no system of organs is entirely free from the effects of the pill, whether the effect is on the biology, the function or the microscopic architecture of bodily cells.

But how important are these effects? Many of the changes for which the pill appears responsible are so small that for most women who take it they may be of no consequence. But the consistency with which these 'trivial' effects are reported means that they should be taken seriously and that certain questions must be answered. If some women's ability to tolerate sugar becomes abnormal when they are taking the pill (as it does), are they therefore liable to develop diabetes, and to any serious extent? If a woman's blood contains more than the usual amount of substances known to precede the formation of blood-clots, does that mean she runs a greater risk than before of dying of thrombo-embolism? Does the fact that the 'profile' of blood-fats in women on the pill begins to resemble the pattern in men, who are at greater risk from disease of the blood vessels and consequently heart disease, mean that they too will become candidates for coronaries in their late forties and fifties?

The dilemma was still the same: the question of how far it was safe to take the pill could not be answered without more research. It was still not known whether it was safe to take the pill for twenty years until twenty years had gone by with a sufficient number of women taking it.

But if the Boston workshop raised more questions than it answered, at least some of the questions were new, and some of the old ones had been given a sharper cutting edge. The huge diversity of the pill's effects was demonstrated in all their bewildering variety: alterations in the breakdown of carbohydrates and blood-fats; increases in the amount of, for instance, iron, copper, insulin and growth hormone circulating in the body; interference with the functions of the liver and the kidney; increased levels of clotting factors in the blood; disturbances suggesting depletion of the body's resources of pyridoxine, or Vitamin B6; contradictory but often profound changes in a woman's mood.

'The effects on a woman's body are fantastic, unbelievable,' said one research worker whom I talked to a few weeks after he had attended the conference. 'We've got to the point where, if you can measure it, the pill can be seen to have an effect on it.' Salhanick points out that it had all been published before – 'if you know where to look for it', he adds laconically. But put together in the pages of a single, compendious volume, it makes a formidable collection.

Some of the conclusions of the conference will be seen in the chapter that follows.

# 5. A High Index of Suspicion

*'The pill is attractive to the public, and to certain sections of the medical profession, because it is simple to administer. This very attraction appears to dull the critical faculties of both patients and some members of the profession. If the reader is unconvinced by this attitude, may I remind him of the thalidomide tragedy?'* –

Mr Patrick Steptoe, writing to the *British Medical Journal*, March 1968

*'In the controversy about the contraceptive pill ... it is just conceivable that some women would opt for a short life and a merry one'* –

Lady Gaitskell, House of Lords, May 1968

Few would have predicted when the oral contraceptive was first introduced in the early sixties that the side-effect which was to cause most concern would be blood clotting. Yet the risk of thrombo-embolism has become the best-known and the most feared of all the pill's adverse reactions.

Thrombo-embolism occurs from the development of a blood-clot, which may break off and impede the normal flow of blood around the body – and it may be fatal. Clotting is a vital property of normal blood. If it were not, we might bleed seriously every time we cut ourselves or had a tooth removed, a risk faced constantly by people with haemophilia, a hereditary condition in which the clotting mechanism works too slowly. Unfortunately, in a vastly greater number of people the reverse is true and their blood clots too readily. And what makes some individuals' blood coagulate unnecessarily and form clots where they are not wanted is one of the most hotly pursued questions in medicine.

A distinction ought to be made, though often it is not, between thrombosis and embolism. A thrombosis is a blood-clot formed in a blood-vessel or one of the cavities of the heart, which stays right where it has formed. An embolus is a clot formed somewhere else which has been carried along by the circulation and become stuck in another blood-vessel which is too narrow to let it through.

The process governing clot formation seems to be different in arteries and veins. Nevertheless, both arterial and venous thrombosis have been attributed to the pill, and there is strong evidence that the pill can cause a thrombus in the deep veins (usually in the legs) which may travel as an embolus to the lungs, and possibly cut off the supply of oxygen to the heart, causing death, or to the brain, leading to a stroke.

Unlike many of the other effects talked about during the discussions at Boston, for instance, the effects of oral contraception on blood circulation have obvious 'bedside' significance. Studying the pill's influence on obscure biochemical pathways is all very well, say those who are unimpressed by such research, but what difference can it make to Mrs Brown, mother of two and three years on the pill, that she is producing fractionally greater amounts than normal (whatever normal may be) of some obscure enzyme? Such matters, said one doctor in New York, are 'the nitty-gritty of biochemistry. Until you can show a doctor they make his patients actually sick, he's not interested.' No such rejoinder could be made when it comes to thrombo-embolic disorders: a woman with a blood-clot is often clinically ill, probably needs hospital treatment, and may even die.

The first published report of a woman developing a blood-clotting disorder while taking the pill came comparatively early, in 1961. She was a forty-year-old nurse, the patient of a family doctor in the small town of Bungay, Suffolk, who had been given 'Enovid', not for contraceptive purposes but because she had a disorder of the uterus which was expected to respond to hormone 'booster' treatment. After several weeks, treatment had to be stopped because she was vomiting severely. Ten days later her left lung was inflamed: X-rays and electro-cardiograms were taken and she was told she had blood clots in both lungs. Happily, she recovered without difficulty and the

doctors' conclusion was that she had had a 'silent' (i.e. symptomless) thrombosis following on the 'dehydration and vomiting caused by "Enovid".'

Similar reports began trickling into the medical journals and
some were of fatal cases. The first fatality in Britain is believed
to have been a twenty-four-year-old Staffordshire woman,
whose unexpected death left her husband with two daughters.
But there was a certain reluctance to take the risk seriously:
after all, it was argued, thrombo-embolism was a known hazard
of pregnancy, women taking the pill were 'pseudo-pregnant',
what else could you expect? An ad hoc committee of the FDA
in America had considered the question in 1963 and concluded
that there was no definite evidence on which to incriminate the
pill in thrombo-embolism. And in 1964, the *British Medical
Journal*'s 'Any Questions?' section gave a comforting answer
to a reader's query on a possible link between blood clotting and
the pill: 'The suspicion that the use of oral contraceptives pre-
disposes to thrombo-embolic disease,' said the journal's expert,
'can no longer be entertained.' Yet entertained it was: and
among others by the Committee on Drug Safety, which was
already collecting statistics, as far as doctors' readiness to volun-
teer the information would allow, on the number of women
taking the pill who suffered from blood clotting conditions.
Within a few months of the *British Medical Journal*'s reassuring advice, Dr Dennis Cahal, Medical Assessor to the Committee, was announcing that recent reports of deaths due to
thrombo-embolism among women on the pill had 'given rise
to some concern'. Reports had reached the committee during
the previous twelve months of sixteen deaths from various
kinds of blood clotting among women on the pill. These, it was
pointed out, were only the deaths which had been reported to
the committee, and there could have been more. It was estimated that throughout the country there were about 400,000
women taking the pill. Out of that number one would have expected thirteen deaths of this kind in women of child-bearing
age; so the figures had not reached statistical significance and it
was too soon to draw any firm conclusions. The committee was
proceeding to collect further information and doctors were

urged to send them details of similar cases they met in the course of practice.

Yet an optimistic view was again taken in 1966 by an expert committee of the World Health Organization. No cause-and-effect relationship, they decided, had been proved between thrombosis and the pill. In the same year, in its first report on the oral contraceptives, the American Food and Drug Administration left the question wide open. They had very little choice, because such figures as they had presented them with an odd paradox. From standard information on the death-rate from clotting in the lungs or brain, occurring with no obvious cause, one would expect that out of the 5 million women then taking the pill in America, eighty-five would die of one of these conditions, pill or no pill. But the EDA had been told of only twenty deaths of that kind among pill-users, and only thirteen of those were 'idiopathic' – that is, with no obvious predisposing cause. Could it be, as the Committee briefly asked themselves, that the pill in some way protected women against thrombo-embolism? The question was asked only to be dismissed: the logical explanation, unfortunately, was that something had gone wrong with the system for reporting the untoward effects of drugs. It was very likely that doctors had simply failed to report deaths to the FDA. It was certainly significant that the number of deaths reported did not show the increase to be expected from the five-fold rise in the number of pill-users from 1962 to 1965.

Altogether it would have been a waste of time to look to the FDA's report of 1966 for much enlightenment on the subject of thrombo-embolism and the pill. It at least revealed how little hard information the FDA had at its disposal and contained the promise that large-scale, carefully designed statistical studies were being set in motion. Otherwise the report was, in the words of one British research worker, 'strictly non-contributory'. Some complacency on the part of the British investigators was understandable, for their own research into the question was by now a good deal further forward. Within months of the FDA's report, the first of a series of papers came from the Medical Research Council's Statistical Research Unit, led by Dr Richard Doll (now Sir Richard Doll, and Regius

Professor of Medicine at Oxford). The first was prepared by an MRC working party, the Drug Safety Committee and the Royal College of General Practitioners. It included the statement that taking the pill did involve 'a slightly increased risk of developing thrombo-embolic disorders'. A woman who took the pill ran a three times greater risk of an embolism in the veins than if she were not taking it. If she became pregnant, the risk was six times greater than normal. Deaths from 'clotting episodes' of one kind or another attributable to the pill among women aged fifteen to forty-four were reckoned to be about three in every 100,000 women per year. (Thirty-eight per cent of women taken to hospital with a clot in the veins had been on the pill. But only eight per cent of 'control' women admitted to hospitals for other reasons had been taking it.)

Should the pill be banned, it was asked? The answer was a firm 'No' from the Minister of Health, Mr Kenneth Robinson: the risk was too slight for such a step. But in April the following year the figures were amplified by a new series of reports. One was an analysis of the death certificates of 334 married women aged twenty to forty-four who had died of an unexpected clotting disorder of the lungs, heart or brain during 1966 in England, Wales or Northern Ireland. The analysis demonstrated a strong relation between the pill and death from an embolism in the lungs or brain, for the women who had died included more contraceptive pill-users than was statistically likely. Out of 100,000 twenty to thirty-year-old women taking the pill, it was concluded, 1.3 would in a given year die of either of the two clotting disorders. Out of 100,000 women aged thirty-five to forty-four, 3.4 could be expected to die. The evidence in respect of coronary thrombosis was less strong: the women who had died of this, it was true, had included more pill-takers than would have been expected from the control group, but the difference was not great enough to be statistically significant.

What about illness which did not end in death? This was answered in another study, published simultaneously by Professor Doll and Dr Martin Vessey. For this, they had worked through the records of all the women in nineteen large general hospitals, in an area of south-east England, who had been brought in with an embolism in the deep veins or lungs. They put aside the case-notes of all those who were not married, those whose records showed there could have been some predisposing cause for the illness (such as pregnancy, a surgical operation, or an accidental injury), those who had passed the menopause, been sterilized, or died, and interviewed the rest. For comparison, the usual controls were chosen, two for each of the affected patients.

Fifty-eight women were interviewed, all aged between sixteen and forty, and all had had their spell in hospital some time in the period 1964 to 1966. Twenty-six of the women had been using the pill during the month before their illness. But of the control patients, who were also interviewed, this was true of ten out of 116 : nine per cent, compared with forty-five per cent in the case of the patients with an embolism.

From these figures, the two medical statisticians concluded, it could be calculated that the risk of hospital admission for embolism of the veins was about nine times greater in women who used oral contraceptives than in those who did not. Looked at in a different way, and based on the available statistics for the extent to which the pill was being used, it could be calculated that one in every two thousand women using oral contraceptives would be taken to hospital each year with a vein embolism, apparently occurring out of the blue. And by comparison, this would happen to one in only twenty thousand women not using the pill.

Doll and Vessey also studied the case records at sixteen hospitals of women suffering from coronary or cerebral thrombosis, clots affecting the heart or the brain. Out of thirteen patients who had survived an unexpected coronary thrombosis, none had been on the pill. But out of the nine women who had had a cerebral thrombosis and survived, four had been using the pill in the month before the illness.

The story told by these papers has since been continued in fresh reports from the same group of doctors. In all of them, scrupulous efforts were made to rule out all possible sources of bias in the statistics. Except that no link has been substantiated between the pill and coronary thrombosis, the later papers have confirmed the conclusions reached in 1968. It has also been shown from scrutinizing official statistics that there has been an increase in the number of young women dying from clotting in the veins. The size of the increase is compatible with the existence of a cause-and-effect relationship between the pill and this condition. (A similar conclusion was reached in the USA from a study of American death statistics.)

Further studies are in the pipeline. One looks at the risk run by women on the pill who have to have a surgical operation. Thrombo-embolism is a known hazard of surgery: therefore it might be supposed that women who take the pill are more vulnerable than others. (If so, they could be well advised to stop taking it in good time before the operation.)

The whole series of papers published so far can be summed up as follows: thirteen out of a million women in their twenties and early thirties who take the pill, and thirty-four out of a million in the late thirties and early forties, can be expected in a given year to die from a blood-clot as a result of taking oral contraceptives; one woman in two thousand on the pill is likely to have to go to hospital with a blood-clotting condition, but only one in twenty thousand of those not on the pill.

The statisticians had at that point found little difference between the effects of the various types of contraceptive pill. (It was not until April 1970 that the Drug Safety Committee was able to declare that if every pill-user in Britain switched to brands with less than 50 microgrammes of oestrogen, the death-rate from pill-induced blood-clots would be cut by half.)

As the researchers in 1968 were careful to point out, one had to remember the risks of pregnancy. These, in some sense, were the alternative to the risks of the pill. Thrombo-embolism is one of the hazards of pregnancy, and indeed only one of a number. The total risk of death from pregnancy and childbirth in Britain was then about 230 in every million women in their twenties and early thirties, and about 580 in every million in the late thirties and early forties.

Though widely praised for the 'elegance' of their design, the British reports of 1968 provoked indignation among some supporters of oral contraceptives, accusations of statistical bias and reminders that, after all, a few dozen dead in one million pill-users of all ages was no cause for panic. It was 'refreshing to know', said one sarcastic reader of the *British Medical Journal* writing from San Francisco, 'despite the "evidence" set forth by the authors that it is apparently still safer to take the pill than to drive your car or to crawl into bed without taking your pill'. Dr Edris Rice-Wray was quoted in a *Medical News* report as stating that she had been on the look-out for adverse effects of pill contraception since the method was first used, had personally treated some twenty thousand women during the previous ten years and had come to the conclusion that 'there are no visible adverse reactions that can be attributed to the pill'. There was absolutely no proof so far, she insisted, that the incidence of any disease was higher among pill-users than in control subjects, and the British data on thrombo-embolism could not be directly applied to women in other countries.

Probably the sharpest critic was the medical director of G. D. Searle, Dr Victor A. Drill, who complained that Doll and Vessey had underestimated the number of times thrombo-embolism occurred in normal women of childbearing age, thus biasing the assessment of comparative risk. Moreover, no excess risk of thrombo-embolism had been shown in fifty-one prospective trials of the pill for which he gave chapter and verse. Later, the FDA pointed out that Drill's rival estimate of the incidence of thrombo-embolism was itself based on seven other assessments, six of which, unlike Doll's and Vessey's, were not limited to cases of idiopathic or 'out-of-the-blue' attacks of the condition, while the one which was so limited produced an estimate only slightly higher than in the British study. As for the fifty-one trials, detecting thrombo-embolism was not their principal aim, and some of them had been done before the risk of thrombo-embolism was widely accepted. The evidence put forward by Drill and his colleague, a Dr D. W. Calhoun, was 'inadequate', the FDA decided, to show that the incidence of thrombo-embolism was either unaffected or reduced by oral contraceptives.

For, however sceptical the pill's supporters were, the FDA

took the British findings seriously. On 28 June 1968, two months after the British results had been published, they sent out one of their infrequent 'Dear Doctor' letters – a letter to every doctor in practice – announcing new labelling requirements for all oral contraceptives, which would include a summary of the new information on thrombo-embolism. 'We urge you,' doctors read, 'to give careful consideration to the information under the various cautionary headings in the labelling.'

Meantime, the American studies were continuing, and in 1969 the first results came out in the FDA's second report on oral contraceptives. The findings from this investigation, headed by Dr Philip E. Sartwell, Professor of Epidemiology at Johns Hopkins University, were substantially in agreement with those of the British group. An FDA 'task force' had carried out a study in five American cities, using the records of women who had been taken to a total of forty-seven different hospitals with some form of unexpected clotting disease. But of 175 women who had been admitted and had survived their illness, seventy-eight had been taking the pill at some time before admission (twelve had been taking it for less than a month – and three of those for less than one week). Out of the same number of control patients, taken to hospital for a variety of other reasons, only thirty-four had been using the pill.

The risk of thrombo-embolism among pill-users was set at 4·4 times that of the non-users. The figure was about half that (a nine times greater risk) arrived at by Doll and Vessey, a difference for which there could be any number of explanations, relating to race, diet or some other social differences. Also, unlike the British studies, there was a suspicion from the American investigation that heavy cigarette-smokers ran a greater risk. And there was clear evidence that the sequential pill regimen, with its greater dosage of oestrogen, was more likely to give rise to thrombo-embolism than the conventional compounds, which were then being taken by eight out of ten American women using oral contraceptives. It was also shown that the risk did not persist after a woman had stopped taking the pill, and continuous use over a long period did not make the risk any greater.

The Chairman of the FDA's Advisory Committee, Professor Louis M. Hellman, reflected in his summary of the report that it had taken eight years from the time of the first reported death from thrombo-embolism among pill-users to establish the relative risk and to confirm a cause-and-effect relationship between clotting and the pill.

One might also reflect that the evidence to this effect had failed in one important way to clarify matters for the ordinary pill user. If the risk had been four or five times greater than it is, it would have been easier to arrive at a decision about the pill's safety. But the risk, as spelled out in most detail by the British investigations, was too small to cause a precipitate flight from the pill to other methods of contraception, yet still big enough to make people uneasy.

One other factor ought to be mentioned. Studies by a Medical Research Council group at St Bartholomew's Hospital suggest that women in blood group A face a higher risk than those in group O: the group calculated that of one million group A women who took the pill for twenty years there would be 689 deaths compared with 221 among a million group O women.

Nevertheless, it is still impossible to define with any accuracy the risk an individual woman runs. If there is reason to suspect she is prone to clotting disease, either from her own medical history or her family's, then she would be foolish to take the pill. But this is not a very reliable guide. A blood clot can form not only unexpectedly but with astonishing rapidity: cases are known, as both the FDA's and the British studies show, where it happened only a few weeks after the victim started on the pill (or even sooner). In January 1971, for instance, the Westminster coroner recorded an open verdict on a nineteen-year-old girl who had died of a lung embolism caused by thrombosis in the pelvic vein. She had been taking a contraceptive pill (a low-oestrogen pill furthermore) for just three weeks.

Bizarre results arising from a pill-induced clot on the brain are occasionally seen at specialist hospitals. A recent report in the *British Medical Journal* described five women, all taking the pill, who developed a minor version of what is popularly known as St Vitus's Dance. Technically known as chorea (the

Greek word for dance), the condition makes its victims perform sudden jerky and uncontrollable movements. One of the worst affected of the five was a forty-year-old woman who had been on oral contraceptives for six days: suddenly when out shopping she noticed it was difficult to keep her left shoe on. Within twenty minutes she began to feel ill: her left arm and leg became stiff and weak and the left side of her face went numb. After a few hours she started to make wild involuntary pumping movements with her left arm, and she could neither eat nor sleep. The symptoms gradually subsided during the next three days. But the one-sided nature of the affliction, the way it began suddenly and gradually faded away, all these, the specialists decided at the National Hospital for Nervous Diseases in London's Queen Square, pointed to some mishap of the circulation, probably a thrombosis. And six days after she had been treated, she suffered a mild stroke.

All the other four patients had had mild chorea at some other time in their lives before they started to take the pill. Once again there is a parallel with pregnancy. Chorea of pregnancy is a very rare complication, usually confined to the first half of a pregnancy and to women who have already had rheumatic fever or chorea at some time in the past: there is a suggestion that rheumatic chorea is caused by some kind of blood-clotting episode.

The investigations in Britain and America had all been concerned with what have been hopefully called the first two 'generations' of oral contraceptive. In fact, as the years went by, the dose of artificial hormones included in the combination pills had been gradually reduced. In particular, the oestrogen content had been lowered: and the oestrogen was the prime suspect in the development of clotting disease.

Hence the bombshell in early December 1969, when it was announced that Britain's Drug Safety Committee was recommending doctors to prescribe, from then on, only pills with a lower oestrogen content. The Committee was understood to possess evidence from statistics of deaths on the pill that formulations containing a higher dose of oestrogen had been implicated in significantly more cases of blood clotting than the pills containing less than 50 microgrammes. Professor Eric Scowen, the Committee's chairman, indicated that if he were responsible for prescribing, he would switch over as soon as possible to the newer, and probably safer varieties of pill.

It meant that about 700,000 British women were now to be advised to change brands. About half the oral contraceptives on the market contained 75 microgrammes (0.075 milligrammes) or more of oestrogen. The rest contained 50 microgrammes. Altogether there were nine low-oestrogen pills available, and two pills with no oestrogen at all, the so-called 'mini-pills': and, as we have seen, they were destined to follow the high-oestrogen pills into limbo within a few weeks.

Tests carried out by a Manchester haematologist, Dr Leon Poller, showed that the danger of blood-clots with progestogen-only pills *was* much reduced. Clotting factors, substances in the blood known to precede clot-formation, increase significantly in women who take the conventional oral contraceptives. In Poller's preliminary trials with 'Normenon' he found not only that there was no rise in the levels of these factors, but also that in women who had been taking a conventional pill, the levels of these factors in their blood tended to return to normal.

Even with the old-fashioned high-oestrogen brands, the risk of thrombo-embolism is not great. Compared with the risk of smoking, driving, pregnancy, and abortion, it no doubt seems to many women a risk worth taking. But – thrombo-embolism is only one of the hazards, and it just happens to be the one which has so far been most accurately measured.

One man who has had a lot to do with the pill from its earliest beginnings, Dr Roy Hertz (now at the Population Council in New York), had this to say: 'On thrombo-embolism I would tell a woman she faces as much danger, if she's on the pill, as of, say, crashing in a jet aircraft. If there were nothing more than that to worry about I would find it an acceptable risk – but one the consumer has every right to know about and not to be kidded about.'

But, Hertz maintains, there *are* other risks: not only over the whole 'vast array' of biochemical changes but specifically, the risk of cancer.

*

The possibility of a cancer scare had been lurking in the wings for several years and it was only a few months after the Boston meeting that it was finally brought into the open.

Publication of the data in question constitutes one of the murkiest and most ill-managed affairs in the whole chequered history of oral contraceptives.

Towards the end of 1968 rumours began to circulate of 'controversial' findings, said to have emerged from a lengthy investigation by a New York pathologist, Dr Myron R. Melamed, from the highly respected Memorial Hospital for Cancer and Allied Diseases. Dr Melamed, who also had an appointment with the Sloane-Kettering Institute for Cancer Research, was believed to have discovered among women taking the pill a significantly higher number of cases of early cancer of the cervix – the narrow passage between the vagina and the womb – compared with women who used a diaphragm. The abnormalities were not cancers in the usually understood sense. They consisted of small alterations in the structure of cells found in the cervix, alterations which have been shown in other investigations to lead on eventually to cancer, though in by no means every case. And, discovered in good time, the abnormalities are curable.

It was not surprising that the rumours had begun to get about, because Dr Melamed had adopted the unusual course of presenting his data to a number of closed scientific and medical meetings in order, apparently, to sound out opinion on certain methodological aspects of his study. Since this had been going on for over a year, it was surprising that the full story of what he had discovered had not yet reached the ear of the public.

At length, in September 1968, a newspaper reporter got wind of a private meeting of a Chapter of the American Cancer Society in Cherry Hill, New Jersey, where Melamed had talked about his survey. Nobody who had been there would discuss what had been said. But one scientist present was reported as saying he did not want to see women 'panicked by sensational news stories'. Far from stifling public interest in the work, such well-meant comments only inflamed it. The panic, however, occurred not among the eight million American women taking the pill, but at the Memorial Hospital, and at Planned Parenthood of New York – the New York branch of Planned Parenthood-World Population. The study, it appeared, had been carried out under the auspices of both these institutions, using money supplied by the US Public Health Service. Both the Memorial Hospital and Planned Parenthood claimed they knew nothing of what was in the report compiled by Dr Melamed. The data were still incomplete, had been under strong criticism from experts, and a lot of work would be needed before they were ready for publication. As speculation grew, Planned Parenthood-World Population thought it necessary to say something to its 164 affiliated organizations, and a telegram was sent to all of them, reassuring them that on the strength of preliminary data there was no need to alter their present policy on the use of oral contraceptives, particularly since all their patients were protected by obligatory cervical smear tests, taken to detect the presence of pre-cancerous cells. In the meantime, the telegram said, the National Medical Committee of Planned Parenthood had called in three independent pathologists to review the pathological material which formed the basis of Dr Melamed's still unpublished results. As soon as Melamed's article was accepted for publication, said Dr George L. Langmyhr, medical director of PP-WP and the man who signed the telegram, 'we will receive a copy of it for assessment in correlation with the findings of the review team' – an observation apparently intended to convey that not all the directors of PP-WP had been allowed to see the disputed article.

But publication, too, was to prove a difficult hurdle. By the time Langmyhr's telegram was speeding on its way to the affiliated organizations all over the world, Melamed's article had been submitted to the *Journal of the American Medical Association*, (JAMA), where it now lay in an ambiguous situation. The first thing that happened to it was that 'revisions' were requested by the editor, Dr John H. Talbott. When they were made, he was said to have found them 'unsatisfactory' and referred the article to another committee of independent experts – this time both pathologists and statisticians. As a result of their comments on Melamed's text, Dr Talbott asked for further changes to be made. Melamed refused to comply. None of this did much to tranquillize the feelings of those who had become caught up in the affair. They included Professor Louis M. Hellman, chairman of the FDA's advisory committee on obstetrics and gynaecology (begetters of the two FDA reports on the pill). Interviewed by a medical newspaper, he declared, 'All of this secrecy is making me uncomfortable. I feel very strongly that there should be no effort on the part of any organized body to withold scientific data. If the investigators want to withhold a study that is their business. But the undue caution with respect to these findings is unfortunate.'

Professor Hellman was not alone in feeling ill-at-ease. Uneasiest of all was Dr Melamed, who stirred the pot with a comment of his own on the second lot of revisions asked for by JAMA. 'We could not agree on the revisions – if that is what they want to call them,' he remarked. 'They had the paper a long time. We made the initial changes that were requested. They couldn't seem to decide what they wanted to do with it.' The suspicion was beginning to be voiced that JAMA was being got at. One report said : 'Some doctors who are privy to behind-the-scenes moves are convinced JAMA is being subjected to tremendous pressures not to publish but decline to say who is doing the pressing.' An intrepid *Medical Tribune* reporter tackled the two biggest drug companies concerned, Syntex and G. D. Searle. Syntex's spokesman said: 'Nobody around here has been in touch with either the authors or with any medical journals about the study.' At G. D. Searle, the reporter was told the company was aware of the paper: 'and we understand that it has been criticized.' Apart from that, the Searle spokesman had no information.

One suggestion from JAMA was that the article should be published – but with the criticisms alongside. Yes, it was an unusual idea, agreed a JAMA spokesman, but not unique. Yes, it was also unusual for an article to be kept in editorial limbo for so long: but Dr Talbott was anxious to avoid appearing to make a hasty decision. 'The editors leaned over backwards in order not to be accused of suppressing the facts,' the JAMA spokesman said. Perhaps they had not leaned over quite far enough: Planned Parenthood were still in the dark at this point about the fate of the article. When brought up to date, Dr Langmyhr remarked stoically that 'there seems to have been a major breakdown in communications between the researchers and JAMA'. He added, 'the situation places everyone in a difficult position.' The communications breakdown affected more people than Melamed and his co-authors: Langmyhr himself had still not seen the manuscript. Neither had any of the other senior staff of PP-WP.

By this time, the substance of Dr Melamed's work was so widely known that in the words of the *Medical Tribune* reporter, it was 'rapidly becoming medicine's best-known work of underground literature'. All the guesswork over its exact contents was finally laid to rest in July 1969 when the article appeared, unexpectedly, not in JAMA, nor in any other of the medical journals allegedly 'itching' to publish it, but in the *British Medical Journal*. The text – final irony – was identical, give or take a comma or two, with the one first submitted to JAMA in the spring of 1968. It had four signatories in addition to Dr Melamed's: three were associated with the Sloane-Kettering Institute and one, Dr Hilliard Dubrow, was an official of Planned Parenthood of New York.

The article, they explained, was the first of two reports to come from a long-term study of cervical cancer in users of oral contraceptives. The second part would need several years for its completion, the authors said, and, from their description, it is likely when it comes to be of considerably more value than the report published by way of a first instalment. It is to consist of a study of the incidence of cancer of the cervix and related abnormalities in matched groups of women known, at the outset, to be free of the disease. One group consists of women using diaphragms, a second group of women using an intra-uterine device, and a third group of women using the pill.

In the meantime, the medical profession was offered the results of a survey of over thirty-four thousand women who had attended one of eleven Planned Parenthood centres for advice on contraception and had chosen either the pill or a diaphragm.

Over twenty-seven thousand had chosen the former, nearly seven thousand the latter, and among the group using the pill there was a small, but statistically significant difference in the number of very early cancers, or 'pre-cancers', when compared with the group who had used the diaphragm. Of the women who had been using oral contraceptives for at least a year at the outset of the survey, sixty-two out of 6,331 were found to have evidence of early cancer. But of 3,874 who used the diaphragm, only sixteen were affected.

Unfortunately, unlike the British studies on thromboembolism, the investigation was far from being clear-cut, and it is not difficult to pick holes in it. Melamed and his colleagues do it themselves. They point out that the difference in the number of pre-cancers between the two groups could be explained in a number of ways. For instance, it has often been suspected that semen or smegma (the glandular secretion from the man's foreskin), or both, may have some influence in causing cancer of the cervix. Lifelong virgins almost never get it, prostitutes frequently do. It is also rare among Jewish women – perhaps, it has been argued, because Jewish men and circumcised. (On the other hand, some researchers have found that Gentile women who admitted to having intercourse with circumcised men had the same incidence of cervical cancer as the rest of the Gentile population.) If semen or smegma are to be implicated in cancer of the cervix, it could be that using a diaphragm offers protection against their cancer-causing potential, if any. Also, there seems to be a class difference. According to one authority, the wives of builders' labourers have thirteen times the death rate from cancer of the cervix found among the wives of doctors, lawyers and clergymen.

Other explanations suggest themselves: it could be that women who use the pill have intercourse more frequently than women who use diaphragms, and hence are more exposed to whatever malign influences this may entail. Altogether, as a venereologist wrote recently to the *British Medical Journal*, 'it is a subject fraught with intriguing postulations and theories, none of which, as yet, seems to have proved conclusive'.

From the practical point of view the long-awaited Melamed

paper made little difference to the status of the pill as a whole. The National Medical Advisory Committee of Planned Parenthood-World Population, having at last had the chance to read the paper they had part-sponsored, gave it as their considered judgement that the pill should remain in 'the medical armamentarium', provided the women who took it were given regular cervical smear tests, as was the rule in their clinics – and provided the FDA continued to give its approval. The FDA had already spoken its mind on the Melamed paper: the data, they had said, neither confirmed nor refuted a cause-and-effect relationship between the pill and cancer of the cervix.

Planned Parenthood also reassured its customers that not all cases of pre-cancerous lesions progressed to full-blown cancer, so far as doctors knew. And in general, it is doubtful whether Melamed's work, and the long-drawn publicity for it which the sponsors' attitude clumsily ensured, caused any significant number of women to stop taking the pill. As Professor Hellman remarked: 'People are much more sophisticated about scientific reporting than they were ten years ago and the pill has had something to do with this. They recognize scare reporting. People have howled wolf too often.' And for all the frightening connotations of the word cancer, it is still for most people, smokers included, a disease that happens to somebody else.

One of the disadvantages of Melamed's investigation was that the women who had formed his group, for all their impressive numbers, were far from ideal as a survey population. The case records forming the backbone of the data were 'service records' from run-of-the mill birth control clinics, never designed to supply information for statistical research of this kind. Precisely the same objection has been made to another time-consuming survey which, like Melamed's, was sponsored by Planned Parenthood and has only been published in an incomplete form. It is being carried out by a group of doctors in Chicago under the leadership of Dr George Wied of Chicago University. Again, large numbers of women are involved: forty thousand in this case. But with the Chicago study, an attempt has been made to find out first of all how prevalent are the suspect 'pre-cancerous' conditions among women in the various susceptible age-groups, and so create a base-line for later comparison. After five years, the investigators found among women taking the pill some eighteen cases in every thousand of cancer '*in situ*' – not high, but higher than normal. But further sifting of the information suggested that this was not altogether a reliable figure and the work is under intensive review.

Nor are Melamed and Wied and their colleagues the only ones to be investigating cervical cancer and the pill. At least – three other studies are either in progress all long-term. One is, yet again, part-sponsored by Planned Parenthood, and is being carried out in California with a clinic population of thirty thousand women. Another is in Britain, under the joint auspices of the Medical Research Council and the Family Planning Association: twenty thousand women are involved, half of them on the pill, half using the diaphragm or an intra-uterine device, and the public will have to wait between ten and fifteen years for this work to be completely finished. Meantime the US Food and Drug Administration is setting up an investigation of its own, in Yugoslavia. Several reasons have been given for this slightly surprising choice. The Yugoslav government is anxious to reduce the high rate of abortion and replace this with wider use of efficient contraceptives. Also, Yugoslav womanhood includes a large number of ethnic and cultural groups: so does the womanhood of America, but in Yugoslavia there is a uniform health service for all, making it what Dr John Schrogie, an FDA official, called 'an excellent research base'. The decision to mount the investigation there rather than anywhere else falls into sharper focus with the information given by Dr Schrogie to an American medical newspaper: 'The Yugoslavs are sitting on a lot of frozen US dollars,' he explained, 'we can't get the money out, so we'll use it there.' The enterprise is being treated with due urgency ('Our priority for this project is tops,' Dr Schrogie said) but only an optimist would look for quick results from this or any of the whole group of investigations – in California, Britain, or Eastern Europe.

It seems then that the whole question of whether the pill does or does not cause cervical cancer has to remain in mid-air for the time being. It is unlikely to come down to earth until there is a solid basis of statistical fact to go on, as incontrovertible as the classic papers on thrombo-embolism, and preferably having passed the scrutiny of a platoon of independent pathologists, able to confirm that the microscopic changes identified in the lining of the cervix really are the kind which could lead to cancer.

One man, however, who probably did not find anything particularly surprising in the flurry over cancer in 1969 was Dr Roy Hertz – the same Dr Hertz who worked on the original synthesis of progestational steroids and was the first to test on animals the norethisterone produced by Djerassi in 1952. He also used the compound as a way of treating women's menstrual difficulties but, he told me in May 1969, 'I did not then and I do not at this time recommend its use for purposes of contraception.' In fact, Hertz has adopted a consistently sceptical attitude towards oral contraception. He observed with sardonic amusement that his paper of 1954 on the progestational effectiveness of the 19-nor steroids used to be cited as a reference in the literature that went with the oral contraceptive packs. When his objections to the pill became more explicit, the reference was quietly dropped. It is impossible, however, for the pill's advocates to ignore him. Not only is he a scientist of considerable standing, with no ideological or religious axe to grind, he was a long-standing member of the FDA's Advisory Committee on Obstetrics and Gynaecology and chairman of the committee's 'task force' on the pill's carcinogenic aspects. In 1970 he was appointed chairman of a newly formed FDA advisory committee on birth control.

Hertz's argument is briefly this. The hormonal system of a woman's body is an extremely delicately balanced mechanism, he says: 'In principle you would hesitate to step up or step down the gears in case the whole mechanism might be upset. It can get upset, as we know – in about ten per cent of couples conception is impossible.' Unless there is some serious clinical problem to make it necessary, it is inappropriate to interfere with this mechanism. Further, for some twenty years it has been known that the oestrogens will lead to cancer in at least five species of animals and in a variety of organs. Therefore

one should at least be alive to the possibility that taking synthetic oestrogens continuously in the form of an oral contraceptive might have the same effect in women. In animals it
takes an average of twenty to thirty per cent of the life span
for oestrogens to lead to malignant tumours. Likewise, nearly
all substances known to cause cancer in human beings have a
latent period of at least ten years, during which there is no
known way of anticipating the growth of a tumour – except by
avoiding exposure to the cancer-producing substance. For instance, X-rays will produce cancer of the skin after about ten
years, while the same time-lag exists with cancer of the scrotum
in chimney sweeps, produced by soot, and cancer of the bone
caused by radioactive paints. There is good reason to believe
that there are close parallels between the species in the way
their bodies react to cancer-causing substances and, by infer-
ence, to the oestrogens.

Any investigation designed to answer the question: Does the
pill cause cancer in women? would have to take into account
not only the long latent period, but also another long period of
risk after the women had stopped taking the pill. 'My guess
would be,' says Hertz, 'that with exposure for five to eight
years you would not feel free of risk for a subsequent decade.'

The organs in which logically one would expect cancer to
develop are the normal 'target' organs for oestrogen – the
breast, the womb, and the cervix. Fortunately, in the case of
the cervix it *is* possible to anticipate the emergence of cancer –
by studying microscopic changes in cervical cells by means of
the so-called Pap smear test (Dr George N. Papanicolaou, a
Greek-born physician, invented the technique). But unfortunately, there are wide differences in the way various investigators interpret the specimens they collect and this is one of the
problems which – behind the scenes – bedevilled the Melamed
survey. Numerous different types of alteration in the cervical
cells have been reported among women taking the pill: they
are grouped roughly together under the heading 'dysplasia',
one of those question-begging medical terms which simply
means abnormality of development. Just how many dysplasias
go on to become 'carcinoma in situ', and just how many of

those become cancer in the normally accepted use of the word – these are matters of controversy.

If Hertz is right, the evidence uncovered by Melamed and Wied, for all its uncertainties and problems of interpretation, could be the first signs of something very serious indeed, a surge in the incidence of cervical cancer and, possibly, other kinds of female cancers which, with millions of women taking the pill, could assume a frightening scale. Perhaps the latent period is coming to an end with the completion of the pill's first full decade, and it may be that we are now about to see the first real effects of its prolonged use. If so, it would be a catastrophe beside which the thalidomide disaster would seem of small account.

Of course, it may not happen. The data collected so far, Hertz has said, are inconclusive, though suggestive enough to demand continuous and comprehensive study of the whole problem. As chairman of the 'Task Force on Carcinogenesis', he said as much in the FDA's second report on oral contraceptives published in August 1969, and pointed out that abnormalities of the cervix did not seem to occur more often with increasing use of the pill: this was not what one would expect if there were a cause-and-effect relationship. Many other points remained unclear. It was also essential to find out how users of the diaphragm differed from pill-users with regard to the age when they first had intercourse and with how many different men, and what the results had been from previous screening for cervical cancer – if any – before the women in each group came under medical surveillance. All these factors could affect the level of prevalence of cervical abnormalities as they had been reported, though none of them had yet been taken into consideration. And if there really was a difference in the current prevalence, and presumably the future incidence, of cervical cancer between women on the pill and women using a diaphragm, was it because the pill was carcinogenic or did the diaphragm have some protective effect?

Uncertain as the position is over cancer of the cervix, it is even more obscure with cancer of the breast. But there are grounds for concern. If women of child-bearing age with metastatic breast cancer have their ovaries removed, so that the body's natural supply of oestrogen is cut off, then in thirty to fifty per cent of them the cancer will regress. In about the same proportion of cases, giving the women extra oestrogen and thus stepping up the supply, makes the cancer worse. But at the same time, in about half the women who develop breast cancer after the menopause, and among a few who develop it in the child-bearing years, giving extra oestrogen has the opposite effect and makes the cancer regress. About all that can be definitely concluded from this is that many breast cancers are influenced by oestrogen. In some the influence is beneficial, in others it is malign. There have been no reports to suggest that taking the pill has led to breast cancer, though there have been reports of possibly significant changes in the underlying tissues of the breast after use of the pill. On the other hand, one of the commonest causes of complaint from the oral contraceptives is that they produce feelings of fullness and tenderness in the breasts, even though the breasts do not actually increase in size.

In the last few years there has been a slight increase in the number of cases of breast cancer in Western countries. Diagnosis has doubtless improved. And there are more women at risk because the population has increased. Pessimists look with suspicion at increasing use of the pill but no one has tested the suspicion statistically. As for cancer of the cervix, the figures are tending to go down, at least in Britain and America, partly no doubt because of better screening programmes, and partly through better hygiene.

It is another story in undeveloped countries, where the facilities for taking and interpreting specimens are either rudimentary or non-existent. The growth of population in such places, however, is an encouragement to cynicism, in the West at least. One American gynaecologist, just back from a visit to India, remarked of the cancer controversy: 'The international aspect is worrying, all right, but if you have a maternal death rate and a population growth rate that are so high, a few extra cases of cervical cancer are neither here nor there. Whether any government could actually say that to its people, I don't know.'

In Britain the most persistent critic of the pill has been an Australian specialist in human metabolism, Professor Victor

Wynn, head of the Alexander Simpson Laboratory for Metabolic Research at St Mary's Hospital, London. Wynn has worked in Britain for over twenty years. He is an outspoken individual whose public pronouncements about the pill in Britain and the USA have done a great deal to arouse the suspicions of doctors and public about oral contraception. Wynn's concern over the subject grew from his study of the pill's effects on how the body handles carbohydrates, and on the pattern of blood fats in women. His research includes a long-term study in which he is following the medical history of over a thousand pill-users, matched with the same number of women using other forms of contraceptive – the largest study of its type in the world.

For long Wynn has argued that in discussions of the pill and its action the emphasis is all wrong. To start with, the chemicals in the pill are much too complex, he says, and the expression 'side-effects' dangerously misleading. If anything is entitled to be described as a side-effect, it is the pill's contraceptive action, he maintains. 'If I said death on the roads was a side-effect of speed that would be nonsense. Death on the roads is an *effect* of motor cars designed to be driven fast. The fact that a car gets out of control when driven at speed is not a side-effect. You can say unwanted effects if you like, that's different. These are steroids – they're not natural substances – with very widespread effects, nine out of ten of which are *not* wanted. That's why I say they are far too complicated.'

Not only are they too complicated, they are not, emphatically not, he says, the same as the natural substances they are supposed to replace. The alterations made by the chemists to produce steroids that were active by mouth resulted in chemicals subtly different from the natural product. Wynn gets impatient at what he regards as glib comparisons between the effects of the two, and at references to a supposed state of 'pseudo-pregnancy' induced by the pill. 'This is a fallacy which is so widespread,' he said at the Boston meeting, 'that it really astonishes me that serious individuals can continue to call the oral contraceptive substances "hormones".'

These views are partly the outcome of a sceptical attitude towards drugs in general. Swallowing medicines in the expectation that they will alleviate pain or abolish some other symptom has become so fixed a habit in the West that it is easy to forget that many of these medicines are extremely powerful chemicals. Although the body may be able to cope with small, irregular doses, chronic dosage over a period of time may have a cumulative effect. One of the most disturbing features of modern medicine, Wynn believes, is the high incidence of drug-induced disease, a type of ailment entitled to be considered a category all on its own. (The Latin-based term 'iatrogenic disease' is ruder: it means doctor-induced.) The true incidence of drug- or doctor-induced illness will probably never be known. But one American investigator found that at the celebrated Johns Hopkins Hospital in Baltimore, during a period of three months, fourteen per cent of the patients receiving medical care also acquired a drug-induced disorder while they were in the hospital. Four per cent of the admissions were in any case due to the effects of drug therapy, and six per cent of the deaths among patients were associated with such effects produced during their stay.

It is even more disquieting that the ill effects of a new drug are frequently not discovered until the drug has been on the market and confidently prescribed for months or even years. Thalidomide is the best-known example, but there are plenty of others, and their effects need not be as obvious, in the end, nor as gross as were the effects of that ill-starred remedy. The whole of human metabolism, with its obscure, often unknown chemical pathways, is a playground for the potent substances on the pharmacist's shelf – a china-shop waiting for a bull to devastate it. But the devastation may be so inconspicuous at first that only long-drawn investigations, with special diets and complicated tests, may be needed to reveal what is going on. Said Professor Wynn, writing in a British medical newspaper: 'The physician, whether he be in general or specialist practice, needs to develop a high index of suspicion about the metabolic effects of drugs, especially if they are intended for administration over long periods. The administration of more than one drug simultaneously increases the risk and demands an even greater search for unwanted metabolic effects.'

In some quarters there has been a certain unwillingness to take these warnings seriously: after all, it has been said, a metabologist is interested in metabolism, he is bound to take such minutiae more seriously than anybody else. This does nothing to diminish the force of Wynn's objections to the pill. As he said to me: 'As someone interested in human metabolism I am against changing metabolic parameters in an unknown way and to achieve a very small result. To produce contraception *is* a relatively small gain, if you also produce a relatively important series of changes in human metabolism.'

Some time ago when I first talked to Professor Wynn in his laboratory at St Mary's Hospital he insisted he was not 'against' the pill. What he was against, he said, was the complacent assumption that the pill was the ideal contraceptive. It was not. Pill contraception, he said in a careful choice of words, was 'one of the most significant medical experiments ever undertaken. It is the job of everyone concerned with humanity to try to promote better understanding of its effects and assist in developing a compound which is effective, safe, and acceptable, as a matter of urgency.'

This, however, was in 1968, and his attitude has hardened since then. The range and diversity of its metabolic effects, as demonstrated in the fifty or more papers delivered at the Boston meeting, create a situation of the utmost seriousness, he says. He has predicted confidently that within the next two or three years, the pill, at least in its present form, will no longer be used: not banned, but just no longer prescribed in any quantity.

In the meantime, he is continuing with his research programme. In this he has been mainly concerned with the way the pill influences the metabolism of carbohydrates and lipids. Carbohydrates are the sugary, starchy substances in foods; lipid is a term that covers a whole range of different classes of fatty, greasy substances. He has found that around seventy-five per cent of otherwise healthy young women taking the contraceptive pill cannot deal with glucose (which is a type of sugar) as efficiently as they should: their carbohydrate metabolism is upset, and tests reveal abnormal quantities of glucose circulating in the blood. An impairment like this is the hall-mark of the diabetic: but in diabetes it is because the individual does not secrete enough insulin, the substance in the pancreas which controls glucose levels in the body.

In over thirteen per cent of his cases he considered that the oral contraceptives had produced a condition chemically indistinguishable from symptomless diabetes. Some women on the pill are also found to have changes in insulin secretion as well: at first, when they have been on the pill for a few months, they may secrete more insulin than normal. It is as though the body is attempting to compensate for the interference, but later, after long continued use, insulin secretion is impaired.

Doctors at Wynn's laboratory have found that the changes brought about by the pill are rather like those found in women who are grossly overweight. Moreover, in women who are already obese, the changes produced by the pill are even more marked.

Related to this is the effect the pill has on the breakdown of lipids, or blood fats. Circulating in the blood are little globules of lipids combined with protein, a so-called lipoprotein complex which is rather different in composition between men and women – until after the menopause, when the pattern, or 'profile', of lipoproteins in women begins to resemble that in men. But with the pill, too, a woman's lipid profile changes to one much closer to the male pattern. Wynn has said that he has found a disturbing number of different changes in the composition of various types of blood-fats in pill users. Pregnancy also causes changes in the lipoprotein pattern, but they are not the same as those caused by oral contraceptives. With the pill, the changes are more like those found in the blood of young men with atherosclerosis: in this condition the arteries begin to be clogged up by yellowish plaques deposited on the inner wall of the arteries, and containing lipid material as well as cholesterol. It is also highly suggestive that after the menopause, the incidence of atherosclerotic disease in women tends to catch up with the incidence among men, leading to the supposition that the normal balance of female hormones affords some kind of protection against atherosclerosis, and that long-term use of the pill may cancel this out.

So now, as well as a risk of thrombo-embolism affecting the veins, the risk of a similar accident in the arteries must apparently be considered – in other words in the other half of the circulatory system.

Several other clues are relevant. In patients with frank diabetes, obesity may be a feature, and there is also a greater risk of atherosclerosis, leading possibly to coronary or cerebral thrombosis. It is also known that if the blood-glucose levels of patients in hospital with coronary thrombosis are tested, many of them are seen to have impaired ability to handle glucose or, in other words, to have 'chemical' diabetes.

The long-term effect of the changes reported from Wynn's unit cannot yet be predicted. Part of the purpose of his research programme is to find out whether the effects become more severe as time goes on. In one of his papers Wynn reports 'striking improvement' in glucose tolerance shortly after discontinuing the pill, but adds the caution that one still cannot say whether this improvement will continue, and it could even be reversed in time. Equally, there are some women in whom the abnormalities last for as long as six months after stopping the pill.

Things would be simpler if there were some way of telling in advance which women out of a hundred normal ones who start taking the pill will develop the kind of effects which have been studied at St Mary's, and at a number of other laboratories, particularly in America. At the University of Miami, Dr William Spellacy has identified certain high-risk groups, women more likely than most to show signs of this symptomless diabetes: he instances older women, those who have had more than two or three babies or whose babies tend to be large and heavy at birth, as well as women who put on weight excessively when they are on the pill, and those with a family history of diabetes.

It has been claimed that the women who develop abnormal sugar metabolism on oral contraceptives are the ones who were abnormal beforehand. But the abnormalities can be produced in women with no previous sign of impairment. It has also been said that by revealing a hidden tendency to diabetes, the pill gives its users an extra bonus: if she discovers she has this tendency a woman can take appropriate steps in good time. When I put this point to Professor Wynn, he answered, 'That's a load of garbage, of course. I mean, do you *want* to bring on a tendency to diabetes?'

On another occasion, Wynn told me: 'We've got a situation where large sections of a healthy female population are taking drugs ... which are reproducing chemical or biochemical changes in the body which doctors are busily trying to prevent happening in the rest of the community. This is a paradox, and one day I think the absurdity of it will be recognized.'

The major problem with the metabolic abnormalities is whether the women who suffer from them will in time develop the kind of clinically obvious diabetes which has to be managed by regular daily injections of insulin for the rest of their lives. The 'chemical' diabetes which can be identified in a proportion of pill-users is not obvious to the person who has it. It is like the type of 'sub-clinical' or 'pre-symptomatic' diabetes which can be discovered in large numbers of healthy-seeming people merely by testing their blood-glucose levels after a meal rich in starch. Numerous random surveys have done just this, suggesting to some that the population as a whole contains vast numbers of undiagnosed diabetics, and to others that the criteria used for diagnosing them need to be re-examined. Investigators' standards of what constitutes 'normal' glucose-tolerance are liable to waver when they discover an alarming percentage of their subjects have more glucose in the blood than they ought to, yet feel perfectly fit and have no other signs of diabetes. (Equally, a woman with abnormalities in the blood-fats may feel perfectly fit and have no overt symptoms of disease.)

Like the pill, pregnancy also brings out a latent tendency to diabetes, or at any rate to abnormal glucose metabolism. In tests carried out by Dr Paul Beck at the University of Colorado, pregnancy proved to be very much more 'diabetogenic' than the oral contraceptives with which he compared it. Although this is in a way reassuring, the difference is again one of time and chronic dosage: pregnancy, after all, lasts for nine months and is not often repeated more than three or four times in a woman's life.

Unfortunately, this is not the only unanswered question. In view of the association between disorders of the blood-glucose and atherosclerosis, who can say whether the millions of women at present taking the pill include a large number heading for arterial disease and a consequent heart attack in early middle age? Some ominous evidence on this score was recently put forward by two doctors from Guy's Hospital, London, who for many years have made a special study of 'sub-clinical' diabetes and its prevalence in the general population. One of their projects is a long-term trial in Bedfordshire, which has been going on since 1962 and which aims among other things to find out exactly how dangerous this 'borderline diabetes' is. And the two specialists, Dr Harry Keen and Dr Richard Jarrett, have found a significantly greater incidence of atherosclerosis among the people with higher blood-glucose levels. 'Two to three times as much arterial disease,' they reported to an atherosclerosis conference in the autumn of 1969, 'is found among people in the top ten to twenty per cent of the total range of blood sugar values as in the rest of the population.' The evidence from the Bedford survey was corroborated by interim results of other surveys in Tecumseh, Michigan, and Framingham, Massachusetts.

Moreover it is still not clear which of the components of the classical pill are responsible for the effects on sugar and fat metabolism, or whether they are due to the progestogen and oestrogen working together. Is there any possibility that a progestogen-only pill might not interfere with metabolism in this way? (There is some evidence that the oestrogenic ingredient is chiefly responsible: and trials carried out with the 'mini-pill', which contained no oestrogen, suggested that this type of oral contraceptive had no effect on carbohydrate and lipid metabolism, though the trials involved only small numbers of women.) And does the disorder get worse the longer a woman takes the pill? Such information as there is on this last point indicates that the abnormalities do become more frequent among pill-users who have been taking oral contraceptives for a long time. When Spellacy carried out tests of sugar-tolerance on women who had been using the pill for more than five years, he found abnormalities in about a quarter of them. After ten years three-quarters of the test results were abnormal. But in this report, there was no information on the women's health before they began taking the pill and there were, said Spellacy, other factors (such as the type of drug used and the test used) which might have upset the results.

The question arises: what practical steps ought to be taken as a result of these findings? It has been advocated that every woman who uses the pill should have regular blood-sugar tests, as she does – in theory – for early signs of cervical cancer. Wynn himself says the repeated investigations needed to check blood-sugar, insulin levels and lipids, are not practicable. Few laboratories have the facilities for it, so that the question of whether such tests should be made routinely becomes a largely academic one. Even so, at a New York seminar not long ago, Spellacy advocated routine sugar-tolerance tests for pill-users. At least once yearly, he said, would seem a reasonable precaution. But it seems likely that the weight of medical opinion is against this. And at the same seminar (sponsored by the drug firm of Eli Lilly, Inc.) what was probably a more popular view was taken by another eminent doctor, who had cooperated with Spellacy in some of his investigations and provided patients for him to study. He was Dr Joseph Goldzieher, of the Southwest Foundation for Research and Education, at San Antonio, Texas. Dr Goldzieher, who was one of those responsible for formulating the first sequential pills, said: 'Suppose we do find a change in carbohydrate metabolism? Can we say that it will harm the patient? All we can say is that a metabolic change has been observed. But this change is not necessarily diabetes or a state leading to it. It may resemble the alterations in carbohydrate metabolism seen in pregnancy. At present we simply do not know what the implications are. And the question has to be studied further.'

Dr Goldzieher was backed up by the chairman of the session, Dr Elizabeth Connell of New York Medical College, who wanted to know: 'What if you take her off the pill and she becomes pregnant? What if she then has repeated pregnancies? Wouldn't that be equally damaging to her carbohydrate metabolism?'

Possibly it would, and as Dr Goldzieher observed, the question has to be studied further. The full story, said Professor Wynn in a report to the *Lancet*, may only become apparent in twenty to thirty years' time. It is a distressingly familiar conclusion, leaving the millions of women who take the pill in the usual unenviable predicament. Meanwhile, some researchers, though not Wynn, believe that a possible clue to what is happening lies in the fact that oestrogens are known to stimulate growth hormone, a pituitary hormone which controls the growth of bone and gains in body-weight. Stress can also step up production of this hormone. And it is known that if growth hormone is injected in big enough quantities it can produce diabetes. And when Spellacy checked the levels of growth hormone in a group of women taking the pill, he indeed found a significant increase, though the group was a small one: thirty-six all told, not all of whom stayed the course.

What other effects the continuous stimulation of growth hormone may have is another matter for conjecture. Again, the comparison with a delicately-engineered and exactly balanced Swiss watch seems appropriate. The turnover of bone cells which proceeds at a controlled rate throughout life is not a process one would lightly interfere with. Yet the pill could be doing just that. Giving the compounds in the oral contraceptive to girls just before puberty speeds up the transformation of cartilage into bone and has the general effect of telescoping the growth of the skeleton which takes place at about this time. Such individuals are, in the phrase of one of the contributors to the Boston conference, 'contraceptive-prone': and a better knowledge of the pill's effects in this respect would be, to put it mildly, welcome. There is also some evidence, though not much, that women who use the pill may have an extra density of bone such as one might expect if too much growth hormone were being produced.

Like thrombo-embolism, sugar metabolism, and a number of other hazards, the effects the pill has on bone growth are duti-

fully included (the duty was imposed in the first place by the
FDA) in the cautionary statements which form part of the oral
contraceptive package literature for doctors. The pill should be
'used judiciously', say the small print warnings, in young
patients whose bone growth is not complete.

Does it all matter? Nobody can be sure – yet. The answer
(and one comes to repeat it with a certain weary resignation)
may not be apparent for another decade at least.

The promotional literature also acknowledges in its deadpan
way the pill's effect on the liver. In view of the widespread
action of the pill, its indiscriminate 'scatter' throughout the
system, it would be surprising if it did not affect the organ
which, besides being the largest in the body, is also the major
site of chemical activity, an extraordinarily complex piece of
biological machinery, controlling a vast number of processes
which can be turned on when necessary: production of bile,
the bitter, yellow fluid important in digestion; manufacture of
fibrinogen, needed to produce fibrin, the basic ingredient in
blood clots; and heparin, a powerful anticoagulant or anti-
clotting agent. Besides being a factory, the liver is also a reposi-
tory: it stores the iron and copper needed to make red blood
corpuscles, it stores sugar in the form of glycogen, and also the
B vitamins. In addition, the liver performs all kinds of chemical
transformations, taking the toxins out of harmful products
made in the intestines and absorbed into the blood; it takes
apart amino-acids and makes urea and uric acid so that they
can be excreted via the kidneys, and is also vitally concerned
with the storage and breakdown of fat. The full story of the
liver's super-versatile role in keeping the metabolism turning
smoothly over has not been established even now, and altogether its intricacies are just the kind which one would expect
to be vulnerable to chronic dosing with synthetic chemicals. In
fact, the liver has been shown to be affected in more ways and
with greater regularity by sex hormones than any other organ
not specifically concerned with reproduction: and their action
on the liver is believed to reach into nearly every biochemical
and physiological system in that organ.

Such investigation as has been done on the effect of the pill on all these functions is inconclusive, as always, and frequently contradictory. Nevertheless, there is general agreement that the pill uncovers any existing weaknesses in the liver's ability to excrete what it manufactures. If the liver's functions are disordered because of an inherited or an acquired condition, the pill can make the disorder worse.

The best-known sign of liver disease is jaundice, the yellow discolouration of the skin which happens when bile cannot escape into the intestines in the usual way, but is absorbed by the blood and dumped in the tissues all over the body. Thus, doctors are warned in the medical literature to look out for cholestatic jaundice (jaundice due to stoppage of bile) as one of the adverse reactions known to occur.

If the pill makes an existing weakness worse, the implication is that it places an extra strain on the liver – a strain which the normal organ can apparently, as a rule, cope with. (Sometimes the normal liver cannot, and the pill may actually bring on jaundice unaided by any existing disorder.) The degree of strain can be measured by various complicated biochemical tests: for instance by injecting into a vein measured quantities of a harmless dye which normally the liver will swiftly remove from the blood, store for a time, and then get rid of. Studying the rate at which the dye disappears from the blood, its storage and excretion, can therefore be a sensitive test of how well the liver is functioning. When doctors use tests like these on women taking oral contraceptives, it is usual to find a significantly higher number of abnormal results among them than among control patients. But some doctors find more than others. The findings are not easy to interpret and it is easy for those who doubt their significance to disparage them on these grounds. Also pregnancy, too, throws a similar strain on the liver, which is felt all the more if the woman already has some liver trouble. On the other hand, one doctor speaking at the Boston workshop (Dr Irwin M. Arias of the Albert Einstein College of Medicine in New York) remarked that oral contraceptives had brought about 'a small epidemic of jaundice' of certain kinds, and indicated that it could be considered normal for the pill to interfere with at least some aspects of the liver's function as a kind of chemical exchange. It was clear, said another speaker, that the 'transport' functions of the liver could be regularly and profoundly upset by a large number of oestrogens as well as by certain synthetic steroid hormones. The mechanism was 'not yet firmly elucidated', 'but the effect undoubtedly finds expression in a substantial number, if not most, women during the course of a normal gestation or during the prolonged use of synthetic sex hormones'.

One of the curiosities of this aspect of the pill is that in the past few years, jaundice appears to have been found more often among pill-users in certain parts of the world. Chile, Finland and the Scandinavian countries in general have more than their share of jaundiced women using oral contraceptives and the Swedish Adverse Drug Reaction Committee decreed as long ago as January 1968 that the statistical link between jaundice and the pill was now proven. No other similar drug-monitoring bodies have made so emphatic a decision.

Although it may be that more exacting standards of measurement are the reason for this discrepancy, another possibility is that in these particular countries some inherited factor is at work. In one series of cases reported from Sweden there were instances where several members of the same family developed jaundice while taking the pill. The woman doctor who is chairman of the Swedish committee, Professor Barbro Westerholm, said recently that drug-induced jaundice or impairment of the liver's functions accounted for seventeen per cent of the reports received by the committee in the four years up to June 1969. Oral contraceptives, she said, 'accounted for a great many of the cases reported'. Half the cases of liver disorder on the pill occurred within three months of starting to take it. And more than half of the women affected were under twenty-five. But they had also found that it was common for the jaundiced women to have had itching or jaundice during earlier pregnancies, and also that these upsets were commoner among their mothers.

Was it the oestrogenic ingredient or the progestogen that was to blame? Professor Westerholm said the evidence on this point was equivocal. There were cases where women had had jaundice after taking progestogen-only drugs, and the same with women who had taken oestrogen only. Her estimate was that perhaps one woman in four thousand using oral contraceptives would develop jaundice, though genetic influences were, she said, of obvious importance.

The capricious results of the genetic lottery are neatly illustrated in the story of two attractive green-eyed auburn-haired sisters in Birmingham, told in a case report from a group of doctors in the city. The two sisters were strikingly alike, and when each was put on the contraceptive pill 'Anovlar', they both began to itch. (Itching is one of the symptoms of jaundice, caused by unwanted substances being deposited in the skin and causing irritation.) One itched so badly that she became almost suicidal, but they had other symptoms as well: diarrhoea, vomiting, and a deeply jaundiced colour. Both, in short, were extremely unwell, and in each case it took some months before their jaundice cleared up: needless to say, neither continued taking the pill. However, it emerged that there was a third sister, quite unlike the first two and in a different blood group. She had been taking the pill too, a slightly different brand of 'Anovlar': she had been on it for two years and had had no noticeable ill-effects.

The case illustrates another aspect of the matter. One of the jaundiced sisters had had three children, and during each of her pregnancies had suffered from severe itching, a symptom probably indicating some degree of liver disorder and usually taken, now, as a sign that the pill should not be prescribed.

Jaundice and itching are not the kind of symptoms that doctors (or patients) can very easily ignore, but this is not the case with the sort of findings which cause suspicion in metabolic laboratories and which require specialist techniques and knowledge to get at them. Not long ago, an Aberdeen anaesthetist interested in liver function took blood samples from the veins of sixty-six women attending a local birth control clinic and found a 'very highly significant fall' in the amounts of a serum-enzyme, 'a very highly significant increase' in one serum-protein and a 'significant' increase in another. So what is liable to be the prescribing doctor's reaction to this news: only one of the sixty-six women had clinically recognizable jaundice, and she was cured after two months' treatment. And besides, the anaesthetist had stressed that one could not infer from his results that liver function was changed either permanently or temporarily to an extent that had any great clinical significance: the changes might be interpreted, he said, as representing a stage before the appearance of outright damage to the liver cells and seizing up of liver function. In any case, the illness suffered by the one woman who was frankly jaundiced was very similar to jaundice of late pregnancy. Everyone could breathe again.

Or could they? Probing into the fine detail of the pill's effects goes on nevertheless, with results that little by little detract from the pill's image as the 'safe, easy, acceptable, *modern* way to plan your family'. More recent research has uncovered another aspect of the pill's action on the liver. One of its effects is to step up the manufacture of a substance called haem. Haem is the Greek word for blood, but in medical terminology it is the word for the iron constituent of haemoglobin, and the substance which gives blood its red colour. Increased production of haem is a characteristic of a somewhat unusual disease called porphyria which is now believed to have been the cause of George III's apparent insanity and to have been inherited by a number of members of the English royal family in the seventeenth, eighteenth and nineteenth centuries. Most of the steroid mixtures used in oral contraceptives raise haem production, apparently by spurring on synthesis of an enzyme necessary for haem to be made. Naturally occurring steroids do the same thing. And so the research does not necessarily mean a sudden increase can be expected in the incidence of porphyria. But following these investigations through leads to another unexpected discovery, and one which could have more disturbing implications. Haem also forms part of another agent in the liver which 'defuses' potentially harmful chemicals – including drugs – breaking them down into a form in which they can be more easily excreted. In the usual way of things a substance which produces extra haem should improve this defusing operation by the liver; but in fact the contraceptive steroids (again, like natural hormones) need defusing too. Thus, if some new load were placed on this defusing system – if, for instance, a woman taking the pill were also given some other drug during an illness – the combined effect of the two might well be troublesome.

To a large extent, this possibility remains no more than a gleam in the eye of a few research-minded doctors. When two chemical pharmacologists at the National Institutes of Health came to review the medical literature a year or so ago, they decided that in spite of the keen interest taken in the problem of how drugs affect unborn and newborn babies, very little information was to be had on drug metabolism during pregnancy, which might have been expected to shed some light on the related problem of taking the pill at the same time as other drugs. Such writing as there had been on the matter of how contraceptive steroids influence drug metabolism was 'inconsistent and difficult to interpret'. As regards pregnancy, the holes in medical knowledge in this respect are not particularly surprising, since giving drugs to pregnant women can hardly be justified by mere experimental curiosity. There is a little evidence that pregnancy slows down the metabolism of some drugs, and there is a certain amount of indirect evidence too, to the same effect, collected from the study of animals. But it is not especially impressive and some of it even sounds faintly comic, with drugged rodents perversely upsetting the expectations of pharmacologists in white coats. Rats about to produce their young, who were given a sleeping drug the day before, slept longer than control rats who were not pregnant, and the effects of the pentobarbital they had been given lasted longer in general. Likewise, rats given 'Enovid' took half as long again to sleep off a different barbiturate than rats who had not had the pill. This uniformity was wrecked, however, by a team of laboratory mice, who had had the same combination of 'Enovid' and hexobarbital. The mice slept for *shorter* times than controls. In one species the pill seemed to slow down drug metabolism, and in the other to speed it up.

So the question founders once more on inadequate knowledge. In practical terms, the research that has been done so far suggests that it would be unwise to predict the effects of a medicinal drug on a woman who was already taking the pill. Or, to put it another way, doctors ought to be sure they know whether Mrs Brown is on the pill when they prescribe phenobarbitone for her insomnia. Whether they always do is a matter for doubt.

Whatever other questions the doctor asks of patients for whom he prescribes oral contraceptives an increasing number of reports point to the advisability of his keeping a check on their general sense of well-being. It is usually believed that the pill is so beneficial as a sexual liberator that switching to it from some old-fashioned form of contraceptive is as good as a course of aphrodisiacs, giving a new boost to libido (or sex drive) and abolishing inhibitions. 'The majority of couples feel that their overall "life situation" improves after beginning oral contraceptives and in many the benefits are profound and far-reaching' – this was the verdict of Dr Malcolm Potts of the International Planned Parenthood Federation in his text-book on contraceptive practice. But against this can be contrasted the observation of the *British Medical Journal* a few weeks later that 'the effect on mood of oestrogen-progestogen mixtures is displacing thrombo-embolic episodes as the focus of disquiet about oral contraceptives.'

The trouble is that the pill's effects on mood are complicated by its effects on intercourse. For most who take it, the pill makes sex more enjoyable: no calculations, no 'messing about with appliances', nothing to get in the way, greater spontaneity – these are the kind of comments made by enthusiastic pill-users who rediscover sex with the aid of synthetic steroids. Small wonder that, as the *British Medical Journal* put it, 'the general tenor of impressionistic reports until recently has been sanguine'.

Yet it should occasion no surprise that the compounds in the pill do affect a woman's state of mind. The natural hormones they are designed to imitate affect mood, after all, often profoundly. Pre-menstrual tension, middle-of-the-month blues, whatever one likes to call it, is an extraordinarily common complaint. Some doctors say twenty-five per cent of women have it, others say a hundred per cent. Anxious, depressed, irritable, mildly confused, unable to sleep and racked by headaches – these descriptions, it would seem from some accounts, fit the majority of western women in the child-bearing years at certain periods of their normal menstrual cycles. And all the evidence points to hormonal factors as the likeliest cause.

On the other hand, in pregnancy, common-or-garden emotional symptoms like these tend to be ironed out: a mother-to-be feels happy, fulfilled and proverbially in a state of blooming health. It has been described as a time when a woman enjoys her body most. By contrast, the post-partum period, immediately after childbirth, is one when the risk of serious psychiatric illness is unusually high. The weepiness, irritability, insomnia and restlessness of this time have been nicknamed 'post-partum blues', and again it is a matter of argument how many women are affected: some say five in a hundred, some say eighty.

The point emphasized by specialists who have studied the problem is that serious emotional upset is likeliest when there are rapid alterations in the levels of hormones circulating in a woman's body. This applies particularly to the days immediately after childbirth and also to the menopause, a notoriously difficult period for women to weather and one which may give rise to all kinds of neurotic symptoms, from outbursts of anger to shoplifting. Thus, taking the pill, and so arranging a regular level of circulating hormones ought to, and in many cases does, do away with the fluctuations in mood that a woman is prone to in the normal way.

Other improvements in a woman's health take place, too, which may or may not be related to her state of mind. In a survey of over 800 women, half of whom were taking oral contraceptives, a Stanford University psychiatrist, Dr Rudolf H. Moos, found that women not using the pill complained significantly more often of symptoms like stomach cramps and 'general aches and pains', as well as being irritable, restless, tense, depressed, unable to concentrate and less able to do their work efficiently. They also had more backache and more trouble with their skin than the women who used the pill. And the pill-takers had slightly shorter menstrual periods on average, with less bleeding and a generally more regular pattern to their monthly cycles.

Nevertheless, with many women who take the pill this physiological harmony does not come about. This was the reply of one woman, a London commercial artist, married with two children, when I asked her how the pill had made her feel:

Awful. I put it down to a feeling like one has in pregnancy where you become a sort of vegetable, and you've got no urge to do anything, apart from mothering. And as I work, I found it very depressing, and also things worried me far more. I just felt very depressed all the time.

Really, it was an emotional thing. But I did put on weight as well, and being in this depressed state of mind made me pick at food more : I was always needing something. I suppose it was the pill. I can't think of anything else, and I certainly felt better since I stopped taking it. I was on the pill for about three years, I should think, but I didn't feel like this all the way through, and not at the beginning. I noticed it particularly during the last year ... I didn't go back to my doctor, I just packed it in. And I did feel better. First I sort of experimented with just taking it and not taking it and then taking it again. And I definitely felt worse when I was taking it ... I'd already tried several brands at the beginning, by the way, and this was the only one that suited me anyway. I had a lot of trouble at the beginning getting on to the right thing.

This, admittedly, is only one woman's story. And yet again, doctors' estimates vary of how many women actually give up taking oral contraceptives because they feel miserable and depressed. But undoubtedly, a lot of women do. In the *Lancet* a little while ago two doctors from the Aberdeen Maternity Hospital wrote, 'At present it is probably true to say that depression and reduced libido associated with the administration of oestrogen-progestogen mixtures cause more women to discontinue oral contraception than any other single cause.' More information comes from the mammoth National Fertility Survey being conducted in America by two eminent sociologists, Dr Charles Westoff and Dr Norman Ryder. In a report on the duration of use of the pill in the United States between 1960 and 1965, they said complaints of 'headache and nervousness' were 'fairly common' among the 285 women in this particular study (approximately one-third of all pill-users) who had used the pill but had changed to something different. Their main reasons for giving up were pregnancy-like reactions, such as gaining weight, tender breasts and nausea, and difficulties with the menstrual cycle (for instance unexpected bleeding, stomach cramps and irregular periods). On the headaches and nervousness, the information the sociologists collected was, they admitted, imprecise, but it seemed that the reports of nervousness reflected irritability and tension rather than anxiety. One woman told an interviewer: 'The first brand of pill I took didn't work – made me nervous.' When questioned about how she knew it was the pill that was having this effect and not something else, she said: 'Yes, I'm sure the pills were the cause of my nervousness because I would always calm down when I went off them, during my period.' A woman whose headaches made her switch to another method of contraception said: 'I had such headaches I could not stand it and it made me so very nervous. I only took them for five days. I had these terrific headaches like my head was going to beat apart. I just couldn't stand it; it works for some people but not for me. Doctor said to stop taking them and maybe I could try them again later but I wouldn't. We are using something else now.'

A certain amount of experimenting is often done to try to find a brand of oral contraceptive which suits the patient best and produces fewer symptoms of this sort. The pills available do have differing emotional effects, it would seem from one of Moos's investigations, in which he found fewer women with symptoms of 'menstrual distress' among a group taking three other combination-type products than in a similar group taking 'Enovid'. But the ones who suffered most from these troubles were a group of women taking sequential pills. They could not concentrate, felt moody, and had more pre-menstrual pain than the other women, and experienced more of the puffiness in the joints that comes from retention of fluid (a complaint common in pregnancy as well as with the pill).

Moos also found what on previous evidence was predictable,

that one in ten of the women who were taking or had taken
the pill had far less menstrual trouble while they were doing so :
but another ten per cent said they had a great deal more (most
of those said they had stopped taking oral contraceptives for
just that reason).

So whatever else can be concluded from the data available, it
is obvious that there are incalculable individual differences in
the way women respond to contraceptive steroids. It is not
unusual for those who hate to hear a word said against the pill
to claim that the unpleasant emotional reactions some women
have are 'all in the mind': the women are worried by newspaper reports or secretly guilty at having suppressed their
natural child-bearing function, at 'going against nature'. The
pill, its protagonists argue, makes a convenient scapegoat for all
kinds of symptoms which either have nothing to do with the
drug or are self-induced. Moos calls this a 'curious asymmetri-
cal hypothesis': if it is 'all suggestion' that makes a woman
feel worse on the pill, why should it not also be for the same
reason when she feels better? Why should improvements in
well-being usually be attributed to the pill, and not the blue
moods, aches and pains suffered by the unlucky ones?

It has been known for the pill to bring on a full-scale psychotic breakdown. One person to whom it happened became a
patient in a North Carolina mental hospital. She was a married
woman of twenty-nine with two children. When the second
child was born she had felt dejected and had had some sleepless
nights, otherwise there was nothing out of the ordinary about
her own personal psychiatric history, though the family history
was suspicious: her father had committed suicide and her
mother had had a severe mental illness. A few weeks after her
second baby was born, the girl was given the contraceptive pill
'Ortho-Novum' : a few more weeks went by, and she began to
feel depressed. Her well-meaning family doctor gave her anti-
depressant tablets but the melancholy grew worse and she
thought she was going to die. She was lethargic, but slept badly,
felt a stranger from her family, and also had severe headaches.
After a few more weeks, the doctors tried something else: psy-
chotherapy. But they also took her off the pill, and the result

(of one or the other) was that she began to feel more cheerful and got on better with her husband.

However, that was not the end of the story. Six months later, relations with her husband had got to the point when she needed to take contraceptive measures again. To save money, she took some of the 'Ortho-Novum' she had at home. This time the effects were swift. Within five days she was back in hospital with 'severe depression and bizarre behaviour' and a condition diagnosed as a type of schizophrenia. It was the beginning of a long period of hospital treatment: she was, of course, taken off the contraceptive pill and in time began to improve. But after being sent home apparently better, she became hallucinated and suicidal, and had impulses to kill her children. She was sent to the State Hospital and by some means not reported managed to get a supply of a different brand of oral contraceptive, 'C-Quens' this time, one of the sequential variety. She felt well taking the oestrogenic series of tablets, but when the time came to take the combination pills, containing a progestogen too (chlormadinone, the progestational drug in 'Normenon'), she soon became once again severely disturbed. Luckily, this episode of derangement was short, and she left hospital in reasonable health after three weeks – having incidentally supplied doctors at the Psychiatry Department of the University of North Carolina with a useful clue, that it was the progestational portion of the combined pill which was probably responsible for her breakdowns.

The same was true of another case reported at the same time: again the patient was on 'C-Quens', again there were suspicious features in her mental history (a breakdown after giving birth to a baby son eight years earlier), and again she became deranged, deluded and also paranoid. But in another case reported in the medical literature, it is possible to find parallels between the type of mental breakdown which very occasionally happens after childbirth and behaviour after withdrawal of the pill. This patient was an intelligent, well-educated Stockholm girl who had become suspicious, jealous and aggressive towards her husband, 'in a way', reported the Swedish psychiatrist who looked after her, 'far exceeding normal limits'. It had all started when she left off taking an oral contraceptive which contained norethisterone: she had done this, it was said, because she was worried about newspaper reports of possible side-effects. Her husband first noticed something wrong when she 'became so unreasonably aggressive at a party that their friends complained about her quite uninhibited choice of words'. The case report goes on to illustrate her bizarre behaviour:

Since then she has become increasingly suspicious and jealous. She has been easily irritated and has frequently kicked and scratched. During these frequent quarrels the patient opened the door so that the neighbours could hear the arguments ... About three weeks after she had been taken ill she ordered an ambulance, giving as her reason that she wished to amuse herself by driving at high speeds round a trotting course ... A couple of days before admission she took a taxi for a 180-mile trip to another town to go to a hair-dresser's. A day later she was found in the street in a snowstorm without overcoat or shoes ...

It is extraordinary that such catastrophic results should follow something which sounds as simple as leaving off taking a drug. And, of course, these are all extraordinary cases – the one or two in a million which demonstrate the remarkable variety of effects the pill has been known to have. At the opposite end of the spectrum of psychiatric illness caused by oral contraceptives is the general feeling of tension, depression and fatigue reported by a number of doctors, but with varying estimates of how widespread these reactions are. 'It is extraordinarily difficult,' complained the British Medical Journal a few years ago, 'to know exactly what the effect of this therapy, if any, is on psychiatric disorders.' Dr Steffan Nordqvist, of the University of Lund, was more positive when he spoke on the subject at the 5th World Congress of Gynaecology and Obstetrics in Sydney, in 1967. His study of the problem had led him to believe hundreds of thousands of women 'may suffer' from neurosis of the type seen in pregnancy. In pregnancy, the symptoms did not last: with the pill, they accumulated. One survey had found between fifteen and eighteen per cent of pill-users had developed neurotic symptoms. And of nearly 350 women aged twenty to forty-five who had started taking the pill in 1964.

thirty-five per cent had stopped because of some kind of disturbance. 'With more than seven million women now taking the pill across the world,' said Dr Nordqvist, 'we have a serious psychiatric problem on our hands.'

One factor that emerged from his work was that depression and other emotional upsets seemed to be more common with the older types of pill, containing higher doses of synthetic steroids, particularly the progestogen content. A similar result came from an investigation by Dr Ellen Grant and Dr John Pryse-Davis in Britain. They discovered that in a group of nearly eight hundred women taking oral contraceptives, depression and loss of sex-drive were more often the result of taking pills with bigger quantities of progestogen. Well over a quarter of the women (twenty-eight per cent) on strongly progestational tablets had these symptoms, and two of the women were so depressed they attempted suicide. Other mood changes they noticed were tiredness, irritability, aggressiveness and (familiar paradox) increased libido. Also, surprisingly enough, they noted that premenstrual tension, which had been a common complaint before the trial started, especially in older women, almost invariably improved.

Probably the most significant discovery they made, from the biochemist's standpoint, concerned the production of a certain enzyme called monoamine oxidase, usually abbreviated to MAO. MAO is known to have some influence on a person's mental state, and substances which actually curb its activity are given to disturbed patients as anti-depressants. These drugs, incidentally, have the strange feature that they react catastrophically with an ingredient in certain types of food: patients on MAO-inhibitors are warned to stay away from a whole list of food and drink, which includes Cheddar cheese, game, Chianti and sliced broad bean pods.

In normal conditions there is a dramatic rise in the activity of MAO in the cells which line the womb during the later stages of the menstrual cycle – the time when less oestrogen is being produced and when women, especially older ones, become depressed, anxious and moody. It is supposed that oestrogen protects women against the depression caused by the MAO enzyme, and therefore that a contraceptive pill containing relatively large amounts of an oestrogen-type substance would have the same effect. Conversely, pills with relatively more progestogen work against this mechanism, and indeed Drs Grant and Pryse-Davis found that in the patients who took such compounds, the activity of MAO in the cells of the womb began about ten days earlier than usual.

Findings like these, tending to incriminate the progestogen in the contraceptive pill, put in a slightly different perspective the British Drug Safety Committee's decision in December 1969 to urge doctors not to prescribe the high-oestrogen pills. Though this may protect women against the risk of blood-clotting, it leaves them exposed to the more common risk of depression – sometimes profound – and other changes in mood.

It has also been discovered that women who take the pill excrete in their urine lower amounts than non-pill-users of certain breakdown products – including one derived from androgen, the male sex hormone – which are also found in lower amounts in women with breast cancer. This emerged from an ambitious, large-scale study of women in Guernsey, directed by doctors at Guy's Hospital and aimed at finding out whether any early warning symptom of breast cancer could be discovered by analysing breakdown products in the urine. (The answer seems to be yes.) Although similarities were found in the urine of women who had the disease and that of women on the pill, the doctors at Guy's stress that their results say nothing about the possibility of any link between the two. More to the point is that the male sex hormone androgen will stimulate sex drive in a woman. Possibly the pill interferes with the normal secretion of androgen, thus causing her interest in sex to wane. In monkeys, too, androgen has been found not only to stimulate sex-drive but to be essential to keeping it at normal. Female monkeys whose androgen-producing glands have been artificially damped down or even removed, can only with difficulty be induced to mate – but their interest in sex can be reawakened by giving them androgen.

Considerations like these led a Birmingham University anatomist recently to speculate whether a solution to the problem of flagging libido on the pill might be to treat women with androgen as well – an idea unlikely to help towards the goal of creating a simpler oral contraceptive, more discriminating in its effects.

In fact, insight of a rather odd kind into the pill's psychological effects comes from investigating how it influences sexual behaviour in monkeys. Monkeys are not human beings, and human sex is a good deal more complicated than primate sex: nevertheless, the research results are clear-cut enough to raise some intriguing questions about what the pill might be doing to sexual relationships between men and women. A fair amount of work on this has been done at the Primate Research Centre in Beckenham, part of the Institute of Psychiatry. From the scientist's point of view, rhesus monkeys copulate in a rather convenient manner: the male monkey mounts the female, thrusts himself in, withdraws and gets off her, then repeats the performance a number of times until he manages a final ejaculatory mount by way of climax. This means that scientists can measure levels of sexual attraction by counting such things as the number of times the male mounts the female and how many thrusts of the pelvis he needs to reach a climax. Another convenient index is grooming behaviour: it has a social significance, too, but the nit-picking and scratching that goes on between male and female monkeys is also part of their sexual relationship and follows a cycle just as their mating activity does.

Removing a female monkey's ovaries wipes out the grooming and mounting rhythms: but oestrogen injections bring them back to normal. Oestrogen injections, when given to female monkeys whose ovaries have not been removed, tend to make them behave according to the usual pattern of the female's mid-cycle: there is more grooming by the males, less on the part of the females.

But the effect of progesterone is rather surprising. The research workers removed the ovaries from female rhesus monkeys, gave them oestrogen injections to bring sexual rhythms back to normal, and then gave them injections of progesterone. This had the effect of suppressing the *male* monkeys' sexual activity: they mounted the females less often and reached a climax less often as well. Some did not reach the point of ejaculation at all. But when the progesterone was withdrawn, everything went back to normal.

If natural hormones had these quite conspicuous effects on the monkey's mating behaviour, it seemed important to find out what effect there might be from synthetic hormones in the contraceptive pill. The scientists gave the female monkeys doses of steroids equivalent to the 'classical' pill and the sequential pill (they had to inject the drugs: the effect is unreliable if monkeys swallow them), and observed the effect no doubt on tenterhooks from behind one-way mirrors. Again the male monkeys' sexual interest appeared to have been considerably damped down by the drugs, with fewer ejaculations, which the males had to work harder to get. What was more, with mixtures that corresponded with the 'classical' pill, the male monkeys' performance became progressively more feeble over a period of six to seven months. With a regimen equivalent to the sequential pill (and so stronger on the oestrogenic side) there was an impairment, but it was not progressive.

The peculiar thing about these findings is that they suggest that in some way the chemicals in the pill, whatever their effect on the females, had somehow got in the way of the males' sexual appetite and, as one might say, put them off their stroke. How had it happened? The answer is far from clear. One suggestion has been that the synthetic steroids somehow upset olfactory 'messages' between the sexes or, in a word, the smell of the female which may be part of her sexual attraction.

In learned articles about this subject Dr Richard Michael, who directed the work at Beckenham, has stressed that drawing conclusions about human behaviour from work on animals is a hazardous business: so it is between all members of the animal kingdom. Although progesterone interferes with mating activity in monkeys, it increases it in mice, rats, guinea-pigs and hamsters. And human sexual behaviour differs from animals' in being as he says 'influenced by so many subtle social and cultural factors'. 'Nevertheless,' Dr Michael has written, 'the possibility should certainly not be overlooked that prolonged medication with these powerful steroids [in the pill] may in time modify human sexual behaviour, in particular that of the male, by influencing the hormonal status of his partner.'

It would not be too fanciful to see in the story of the Beckenham monkeys an explanation for the occasional rare cases of impotence in men whose wives take the pill. Psychiatrists have concluded from this symptom that some husbands, and not only those who become impotent, feel obscure resentment and inadequacy when unusual demands are made on their sexuality. But it is just possible that an equally obscure biochemical disharmony lies at the bottom of it. If the husband's sex-drive were to peter out simultaneously with an increase in his wife's libido this could make matters even worse.

For the time being, however, the question remains highly theoretical and unlikely to create major difficulties or be a serious reason for discontinuing oral contraceptives. Almost as remote, for all the excitement with which it was reported, must be the risk described in all seriousness recently in a London newspaper: that ageing, out-of-condition men, whose wives take the pill and so become 'too demanding', risk a fatal heart attack through excessive sexual exertion. Far worse, said the report, for the middle-aged man with a mistress as well as a wife – and both on the pill. 'He would really be under a strain,' agreed an anonymous doctor, who lent some much-needed credence to the story by pointing out that deaths from heart disease were increasing. ('The pill is a definite suspect,' he said.)

Whatever other needless fears this story provoked, it no doubt reinforced the general assumption that the pill is a sexually liberating force, which abolishes fears and inhibitions, leaving nothing in the way of full and natural enjoyment of erotic pleasure. This assumption has been fortified by clever advertising, as well as by hearsay stemming from the perfectly genuine improvement in the sex lives of thousands of couples. But for the not inconsiderable number of women who, equally genuinely and for medically understandable reasons, become depressed and anxious on the pill, the enviable experiences of other women could add to their troubles. Fear of pregnancy may have gone, to be replaced by fears of sexual inadequacy: the fear that there must be something wrong with them if they cannot enjoy sex as one is supposed to on the pill. But it does not follow that they are neurotic or inadequate. It is not necessarily 'nerves' or that they are 'no good at sex'. It may well be their body chemistry that is being affected.

Headache has been listed under the 'trivial or annoying' reactions to the pill, which would itself annoy women whose headaches with oral contraceptives are severe. Many 'pill headaches' probably have a psychological origin, which does not make them any less disagreeable to the individual who has them: only to the ignorant does 'psychological' equal 'imaginary'. And they can also be another manifestation of the pill's action on the blood circulation.

Headaches on the pill come in all varieties of severity, from the vaguely uncomfortable to the barely tolerable, and including something no different from full-scale migraine.

Migraine is a puzzling disorder and its precise cause is unknown. 'Cure' is not a word many neurologists would use in front of people who suffer from it: the best that can be hoped for is that the attacks (which can be hellishly frequent, sometimes two or three a week) will gradually fade away and never come back, as is sometimes the case. In the meantime, doctors can alleviate the symptoms with drugs. The list of symptoms is dominated by the headache, which sufferers describe in such terms as 'cruel', 'fierce', blinding', 'piercing' and 'throbbing'. The pain is concentrated in the temples, the eyes seem to bulge like billiard balls and it makes you want to lie down in a dark room until it has gone, which may not be for forty-eight hours or more. The victim also feels sick, and often vomits. And the whole attack is usually preceded by warning symptoms: sometimes a paradoxical and, in the circumstances, quite unjustifiable feeling of optimism, but more often weird visual disturbances, with blind spots and flickering lights in a zig-zag pattern. These are known as fortification spectra, because the shape looks a little like the regular up-and-down pattern of castle battlements.

This is the kind of headache that can in some cases be duplicated by the pill. And the event which causes this collection of symptoms is generally believed to be a spasm in the bloodvessels near the brain, which first squeeze tight, then dilate as though to compensate for the constriction. Curiously enough certain foods bring on an attack in some people, and they learn to avoid such things as chocolate, cocoa, and some kinds of cheese. Intriguingly, there is some similarity between this list and the foods which have to be avoided by patients who are taking the MAO-inhibiting drugs, mentioned earlier. The supposition advanced by some research workers is that MAO-inhibitors lead, by obscure biochemical pathways, to substances called pressor amines entering the blood stream and resulting in high blood pressure and headache.

Among the incidents which can bring on an attack of migraine is the beginning of a woman's menstrual bleeding, and migraine is something like one and a half times as common in women as it is in men. It is also a common observation that a woman's migraine will often disappear, or change character, after the menopause. Sometimes it improves when she is pregnant, but comes back: it has been known for the first new attack to start within two or three hours of the baby being born. For these reasons, as early as the nineteen-forties progesterone was being used to treat migraine by injection, and some success was achieved.

All this makes it less unexpected that headache as well as true migraine should be a common side-effect with the pill. Oddly enough women who do get severe headache when taking the pill find as a rule that the attacks come on between one month's course of tablets and the next: this suggests that the headaches may be the result of withdrawing the synthetic hormones, just as migraine occurring at the end of the month could be caused by an abrupt fall in the levels of natural hormones circulating in the body. It could also explain why progesterone can make an effective treatment, by maintaining the supply of the hormone at a constant level instead of subjecting the body to a sudden change.

As usual, there are conflicting estimates of how often head-aches of all kinds occur when a woman is on the pill, and things are complicated by the difference between various types of pill as far as their effect on headache is concerned. Nor is it easy to be sure how many women in a given survey were having 'simple headache' (though headache is seldom simple), or true migraine, with its classic triad of symptoms: frontal headache, nausea, and visual disturbance. Dr Ellen Grant, of the Council for the Investigation of Fertility Control (the research arm of the British Family Planning Association), describes the typical 'pill headache' as follows: it comes on soon after starting to take oral contraceptives, usually happens in the intervals be-tween rounds of tablets, but in a few women goes on continu-ously. Sometimes they feel very sick and perhaps they vomit. Some women feel dizzy and have hot flushes, and some have the blind spots and flickering shapes that come before 'ordin-ary' migraine, not caused by the pill. In one or two cases the symptoms become more serious with several years of pill-taking, and can lead to palpitations, pains in the chest, high blood pressure and even minor damage to the brain: but these side-effects generally improve if the woman stops taking the pill.

Meanwhile, one group of doctors reported headaches in eleven per cent of 166 women, another found a 3·2 per cent incidence. Dr Edris Rice-Wray said it varied between 1·2 per cent and 6·2 per cent according to the drug used, and Dr Aviva Wiseman of the Slough (Bucks) Family Planning Centre reported between three and twelve per cent. Two Swedish doc-tors in 1968 said that as many as thirty per cent of a group of patients had headaches in the first cycle, but less than ten per cent after that. And Dr Joy West, of the Family Planning Asso-ciation, found an incidence of 19·9 per cent.

When she studied a group of five hundred women, from the case-records of various FPA clinics, Dr Ellen Grant reported that the incidence of headache among them varied from eight to as many as sixty per cent, depending once again on the brand of pill they had been taking: altogether sixteen different varieties were represented in her list. The attacks, she said, seemed to be under the control of very subtle changes in the ratio of oestrogen and progestogen in the mixture, not to mention the individual susceptibility of each of the women. She had also found that the women who had the headaches tended also to have excessive development of the small blood vessels of the lining of the womb. And it was tempting to suggest, mused the *British Medical Journal*, that these changes were typical of effects on the blood-vessels elsewhere in the body, but so far undiscovered.

Most of the women whose case-records were studied for the purposes of her report had found the pill so efficient and beneficial, said Dr Grant, that few of them gave it up unless they had a lot to complain about. Headache was the commonest of their complaints (followed by changes in mood, changes in the veins, irregular periods and gaining weight). The headache, commented the *British Medical Journal*, might be 'a small price to pay for freedom from the tyranny of fertility'. But considering the large number of British women taking the pill, and that with some brands the incidence of headache was over fifty per cent, 'the total burden of pain is considerable'. Rather more cheerfully, the editorial-writer added: 'That so many women are willing to bear that burden is at once a tribute to the effectiveness of oral contraceptives and an indication of the widespread need for such agents.'

It is well known that many patients, on being questioned, will give the answers they think the doctor wants. In Texas, Dr Joseph Goldzieher discovered a fourteen-fold variation in the reported incidence of headache between various clinics. It was even more when nausea was the subject of questioning, and that was when only *one* pill formulation was being evaluated. The variation from one clinic to another, says Goldzieher, was beyond the difference to be expected from mere random sampling, and the explanation must lie, he thinks, in a combination of differences between various groups of patients *and* different techniques of questioning used in each of the family planning centres. At Slough, Dr Aviva Wiseman says her own data make it clear that the discrepancy goes beyond even the difference between groups of patients and between one formulation and another. The incidence of headache on the pill, agrees Dr Joy West, varies from doctor to doctor and often partly reflects the doctor's own attitude towards oral contraceptives. 'Many women,' she says, 'accept headaches as commonplace, and will not mention them unless specific inquiry is made; others will obediently produce a symptom that is suggested to them.' In the nature of things, deciding on the severity of headache is a subjective affair, she reasons, and the best guide is how many women find their pill headaches so disabling that they give up taking the pill altogether. Of over a thousand women who had been prescribed the pill at Croydon from 1962 to 1967, 19·9 per cent had complained of headache; 12·5 per cent of them gave up the pill for this reason. A significant proportion of those had had migraine in the family or had had it themselves, and measurements of electrical signals from the brain showed abnormalities which suggested latent migraine, Dr West said in a letter to the *British Medical Journal*. Those abnormalities were still there when they took electro-encephalograms of some of the women who had *stopped* taking the pill. Thus, the pill had only brought to the surface something that was already there – again, challenging the body's reserves and exploiting an existing weakness.

At an international symposium run recently by the Migraine Trust, a Paris neuro-psychiatrist, Dr Roger Pluvinage, gave details of a series of his patients which illustrate more of the pill's apparently paradoxical effects. Some of Pluvinage's patients had had migraine before they started to use oral contraceptives; others had never had it until the pill gave it to them. If they had had it before, in most cases the pill made it worse, the attacks being more frequent and the pain greater. But in many of these cases, matters could be much improved by switching to a different brand of pill (formulations low on oestrogen generally seemed to be the best). And such was the benefit from the changeover that the doctors were able to get better results when they treated the women with standard anti-migraine drugs, even though in the past these had had little effect. Some of the other women who had never had migraine before could be helped by switching to a different oral contraceptive and being given tranquillizers, so landing in the slightly crazy situation where the patient has to be given a second drug to counteract the effects of the first, the first one, in this case, being a 'social' drug, not a medicine.

Pluvinage believes a fair proportion of all the patients – just under one-third – had some emotional instability. It is, of course, well-known that migraine tends to affect the nervous, introspective type of individual and some say, reassuringly, the more sensitive and intelligent. However that may be, Pluvinage's psychiatric investigations uncovered a variety of secret fears: anxiety over what the pill might do to a subsequent pregnancy, guilty feelings over what friends, the family, or the priest might say, and in one case, apparently a castration complex. Often, the fact that the wife was taking the pill did disagreeable things to a married couple's relationship, bringing to the surface a fear that the husband might have affairs with other women, or resentment that he should have suggested, as was sometimes the case, a contraceptive method which the wife obscurely felt unnatural and possibly dangerous. And these hidden anxieties expressed themselves as headaches and migraine.

It could be maintained that the pill had been beneficial in conjuring forth these secret fears and providing an opportunity for the woman to have the appropriate treatment, which frequently turned out to be tranquillizers. But the fact remains that in a proportion of pill-users, and it is not clear how many, something is happening in the blood vessels in the head which ought not to be happening, and would not be happening if the patient were not taking an oral contraceptive. Though it is unwise to assume too much from a small number of cases, an incident at a neurological meeting in 1967 which concerned nine women, all on the pill, gives food for thought. At this meeting, organized by the American Academy of Neurology in San Francisco, three neurologists from Cleveland gave a report on the nine patients, all aged between twenty-three and forty-five, and all of whom had developed some degree of brain damage after taking oral contraceptives. The damage was not necessarily serious, though it must certainly have scared them:

the case-histories included temporary partial blindness, impaired speech and permanent paralysis of one side. Four of the women had had strokes. In each case, the woman had had migraine while taking oral contraceptives. The oldest woman studied, aged forty-five, had had migraine before taking the pill. She had started to complain of headache behind the left eye, which grew worse and worse. Then her speech became incoherent and she found that on her right side she was less sensitive to pain. Once she was taken off the pill, she began to improve. Less fortunate was a woman of thirty-one. She had not had headaches before. But a few weeks after taking the pill, she began to have them on both sides of her forehead. The pain grew worse and she began to have blind spots in her vision. Her speech became progressively more slurred and she had muscular weakness down her right side. She stopped taking the pill, but was left with a permanent speech impairment.

Dr John H. Gardner, the senior neurologist of the group who presented the report to the meeting, asked how many members of his audience of two hundred specialists had seen similar incidents among women taking the pill who had developed migraine. 'About two-thirds raised their hands,' reported the Washington correspondent of the *New Scientist*. 'Stroke,' said Dr Gardner, 'is a very rare complication of naturally-occurring pregnancy. But in the "chemical pregnancy" induced for contraception it is the synthetic hormones – more potent than the natural hormones – which seem to cause the trouble. It may be that migraine is either precipitated or aggravated by the cyclical changes which these "progesterones" induce.' With the migraine so aggravated, he continued, during that period of an attack when the blood vessels are constricted, not enough blood gets through to certain parts of the brain. 'This may be the cause,' Dr Gardner said, 'of the focal neurological symptoms – numbness, temporary paralysis, impaired vision – which we have observed with migraine in women taking the pill. If the migraine increases, as it did in our patients, there comes a critical point at which the brain is not getting enough blood. And then a stroke – often mild, but sometimes severe – will develop.'

The number of patients involved might be small, he said. But 'vascular headache', accompanied by signs of specific neurological damage, should always be a warning to discontinue taking the pill. It is a slim chance, but it exists, that an attack of migraine caused by oral contraceptives could herald a stroke.

But an extra dimension is given to this problem by yet another of the pill's actions, or possibly another manifestation of the same one, and which has only lately begun to come to the surface: the risk of hypertension, or raised blood pressure. Random cases have been appearing in the medical journals for some time. Four years ago a Canadian doctor reported a patient who had had high blood pressure during the seventh month of her pregnancy: her condition was perfectly normal in every other respect. After she had had her baby, she was put on 'Enovid'. Two months later she went back to her doctor with headaches and visual disturbances. This time her blood pressure was even higher. She stopped taking the pill. And within a few weeks her blood pressure had returned to normal and she had no headache. She did complain of difficulty in passing water but her doctor discovered an infection of the urinary tract which he treated successfully with antibiotics. A letter from G. D. Searle's medical department stated that the reported incidence of high blood pressure among women taking the pill paralleled the numbers in women generally, and suggested that some women particularly likely to develop high blood pressure in late pregnancy might also develop it when they took drugs containing oestrogen.

This no doubt set minds at rest. But isolated cases continued to reach the journals and there is now a strong suspicion among doctors that the pill sends up the blood pressure among certain susceptible women. So much so that a group of doctors at the Stanford Medical Centre in Palo Alto, California, have described hypertension due to oral contraceptives as 'at the present time, the most frequently encountered, curable form of high blood pressure in our suburban Californian community'. Curable, because the condition can be simply remedied by finding a different method of contraception. But no large-scale, carefully controlled studies have been carried out as yet which could define the association between hypertension and the pill.

Professor James W. Wood of the Medical School of the University of North Carolina, said to the Boston meeting of December 1969: 'The information to date is largely anecdotal. That there is an association, however, appears to be widely accepted among practising physicians.'

Most women taking the pill will *not* have hypertension, that much is clear. How many will, is not yet known: the only possible answer at present is 'some'. Coincidence, perhaps; but in a number of the cases reported, as the Stanford doctors implied, the effects were reversed and blood pressure returned to normal when the woman stopped taking oral contraceptives. A group of doctors from Columbia University Department of Medicine studied eleven women who had come into the Presbyterian Hospital, New York, with hypertension. All had been using the pill. When they stopped, the symptoms of hypertension disappeared in three of them and in another three it was much improved. One of each group then started taking the pill again: back came the hypertension symptoms. Five out of the eleven had had hypertension before they ever started to take oral contraceptives, and in one of these women, curiously, taking her off the pill seemed to cure her high blood pressure completely. Her blood pressure went down and had stayed down when she was seen again a year afterwards.

But the evidence to support a cause-and-effect relationship is more than circumstantial. Closer examination of these women, and of patients in other centres, showed that they had abnormalities in blood constituents which could account for the increased blood pressure. These abnormalities have to do with the body's normal system for controlling blood pressure: an enzyme called renin is released from the kidney when pressure falls too low. It 'digests' a protein substance in the plasma called hypertensinogen to produce a very potent pressure-raising agent called hypertensin. The quantities of these substances in the blood can be measured by various metabolic tests. It has been found that taking oral contraceptives can increase the activity of renin in the plasma, leading to increased amounts of hypertensin in the blood. The doctors at Stanford Medical Centre reported on eighty patients with hypertension, a randomly chosen group, though thirteen of them proved to be taking the pill. Not all of the women had any noticeable symptoms, but among the things patients complained of were headaches and dizziness. When they were taken off the pill, blood pressure in all but one case either returned to normal or improved. But the doctors also found a three to five-fold increase in the concentration of the protein hypertensinogen, and on average twice the normal amount of hypertensin, the pressure-raising substance derived from it.

How this effect is produced is not yet known. The component of the pill which is responsible has not yet been identified either, but the common suspicion is that the oestrogenic ingredient is to blame. It also seems likely that as a rule the pill does not increase the amount of renin, but only increases the amount of hypertensinogen ready to be digested into hypertensin, an event which somehow excites the renin to greater activity and accelerated production of pressure-raising substance. But in its versatile way, the pill can in some cases, it seems, raise the levels of renin too, by a different process.

What is going on to bring about these alterations from normal remains a mystery for the time being. It is some small consolation that specialists have remarked that the pill's effects in this respect may throw new light on how and why hypertension should develop in people who are not taking oral contraceptives.

It is generally assumed that one thing the pill will not do is interfere with a woman's ability to bear children once she stops taking it.

Rock's early experiments in Boston, when he gave progesterone to his infertile patients, then withdrew it, were a great success. They established the existence of a 'rebound' effect through which the women became more fertile than ever after their reproductive machinery had been held in check for a few months.

Subsequent research seemed to confirm this. Dr Joseph Goldzieher reported in 1964 that in a group of women who had discontinued the use of the contraceptive pill 'Ortho-Novum', the pregnancy rate in the first cycle was sixty-two per cent. This compares with a figure of thirty-four per cent in women who had stopped using other methods of contraception. It is an impressive figure, though it has to be borne in mind that many of these women had stopped using the pill because they wanted to become pregnant. One would therefore expect the number of pregnancies to be high.

Gynaecologists still use the pill in the way Rock used natural progesterone in the mid-fifties, to stimulate the rebound phenomenon after a few months' use of the drug. Nevertheless, there is reason to suspect that long-term use of the pill may have quite the contrary result. A recent report in a British medical newspaper, *Medical News-Tribune*, spoke of 'a growing clinical impression that instead of the once favoured rebound hyperfertility there may actually be a rebound infertility'. According to the paper's account, the gynaecologist Mr Stuart Steele considered that there were two groups of women who missed their periods after discontinuing the pill: those whose periods did not return for two or three months; and a 'very worrying' group for whom the return of normal menstruation was delayed for much longer.

The 'clinical impression' referred to in *Medical News-Tribune*'s story was supported by the observations of several doctors, one of whom, an unnamed woman endocrine specialist in London, was quoted as saying, 'We must not wait until we have a sterile generation before the danger of infertility is acknowledged.'

In fact there is already some evidence to bear out these suspicions. As long ago as 1966 Dr Rodney P. Shearman of Sydney University, Australia, published a preliminary paper in which he reported having studied eighty-six women whose menstrual periods had ceased for no apparent reason. Nine of these women had been using oral contraceptives. It might, he admitted, have been a coincidence: the amenorrhoea, to give it its technical name, might have arisen from other causes which had been masked by use of the pill. But there were several reasons why the former pill-users did not fit in with the other women to form a neat and tidy series of patients. For instance, the others included women for whom there was some likely-sounding explanation for the amenorrhoea, women who had menstruated regularly until they had undergone some important change in their family lives, or had decided to go on a diet; they also included women who had always had irregular periods. This was not so with the women who had been using oral contraceptives. Laboratory tests showed that the pill-users' ovaries were potentially able to produce ova, suggesting that the cause of the trouble lay in the hypothalamus or the pituitary, respectively the part of the brain and the gland with overall control of sex hormone production. Dr Shearman reasoned that it was possible that prolonged interference with the function of those glands might very occasionally disrupt the normal hormone cycle – just as, very rarely, normal pregnancy could. 'We cannot yet be certain,' Dr Shearman said, 'whether the association (between amenorrhoea and the pill) is causal or casual, and we present our findings to stimulate future clarification.'

Two gynaecologists from San José, California, also noticed amenorrhoea and infertility among women who had been using the pill: they told a medical meeting in 1966 of seventeen women who had come to their notice, some of whom, having left off taking oral contraceptives, had not menstruated for a year. They had been using the pill for periods varying between two-and-a-half months to four years. The two doctors, Dr James Whitelaw and Dr Vincent F. Nola, said they had found abnormalities in the wombs of several of their patients and severe atrophy in a few. But they agreed that the effect might be temporary, and added that, in any case, some of the women had originally taken the pill because they were infertile. When Dr John Rock was asked to comment on these findings, reported at a meeting of the American Academy of General Practice in Boston, he was clearly unimpressed: the conditions the two San José doctors had seen, he said, could be observed in patients who had not taken steroids. Another pill expert, Dr Robert Greenblatt, of Augusta, Georgia, was much more scathing: 'The report was misleading, the inconsistencies are glaring, the choice of histological description, unfortunate.'

However, two years later Dr Shearman was again reporting prolonged infertility after a spell on oral contraceptives. He had now seen, he reported to *The Lancet* in February 1968, twenty-two patients who had remained infertile for at least twelve months after stopping the pill. There was still not enough evidence, he thought, to clinch the connection between the two, and it was reassuring that in all except one of the twenty-two women, who was having a premature menopause, the ovaries were capable of responding to treatment. He had treated twelve of the women with the 'fertility drug' clomiphene, and eleven of them had ovulated and six had conceived (one had twins). This favourable response, Shearman indicated, was considerably higher than one would have expected in women who were failing to menstruate.

These reports began to stiffen doctors' doubts. 'In the light of our present knowledge,' said the gynaecologist Mr Patrick Steptoe in a letter to the *British Medical Journal* in March 1968, 'it appears to me to be dangerous to give patients who have not proved their fertility oral contraceptive pills for more than a very short period of time, such as might be given for the treatment of menstrual disturbances and dysmenorrhoea.' Steptoe, well-known for some brave-new-worldish research on the fertilization of human ova outside the womb, has carried out a number of examinations of the ovaries of patients who had been taking the pill for three years or more. Some of these, like Shearman's patients, had not menstruated for at least a year and there were several abnormalities in the cells of their ovaries. There is a growing amount of evidence, Steptoe says, to link the pill with infertility. 'The long-term use of these pills carries with it a definite danger of inducing irreversible sterility.'

This was not what the World Health Organization study group on the progestogens had decided in 1966, and the London endocrinologist Dr Gerald Swyer was quick to write to the *British Medical Journal* to say so. He considered Steptoe's findings in the ovaries of pill-users 'not original' (one of the most censorious accusations in everyday medical controversy), and the implication that they represented damage to the ovaries was not borne out by his own statement that many of the women who did not ovulate could be induced to do so by the use of drugs. Probably, Swyer went on, the amenorrhoea which sometimes happened after discontinuing the pill ('in a small but at present undetermined proportion of women') was due to a disturbance of the mechanism for producing the appropriate hormones from the hypothalamus – 'a condition', said Swyer, 'which arises spontaneously often enough'. Steptoe had drawn a parallel between the pill and thalidomide: Swyer thought this 'irrelevant and even irresponsible'.

It remains to be seen which of them is right, and follow-up investigations could also throw light on a related question, which has worried women since the early days of pill contraception: can the pill affect future babies? If it does, nobody has yet been able to prove it, and there is no evidence of any 'clinical impression' to this effect. On the other hand, it is extraordinary that so far no large-scale series of patients has been studied to see what effect the pill might have on later pregnancies. That has been the complaint of a Canadian research worker, Dr David N. Carr, who is Associate Professor of Anatomy at McMaster University, Hamilton, Ontario. At a symposium on birth defects held at Niagara Falls in the autumn of 1969 Dr Carr said: 'What isn't comforting is that thousands of children are being born after the pill, but there is no large series on them. This is a very bad situation. There may be medications, not just hormones, but things like LSD for instance, that leave after-effects. We should look at the offspring of women who have been on medications.' What he urged his listeners to do was 'corner the market in abortuses' if they had any influence with nearby maternity units. The babies who were aborted constituted what he called 'a gold mine of information which now goes down the drain'.

More comforting, however, was the fact that Carr's researches gave no indication of abnormal numbers of defective children being born to women who had been on the pill. But he believed the pill might slightly increase the risk of an abortion occurring spontaneously. Possibly, he reasons, the pill does cause defects in the unborn child, but in some way the mother's body can 'recognize' them and reject them. Animals are apparently able to do this: Carr describes them as 'super-efficient' at it. 'Their abnormal birth-rate,' he says, 'is much lower than humans', even at term. But they are so clever at getting rid of such abnormal offspring by reabsorption that it is difficult to detect their mechanism.' If one could detect it, it might lead to a method of making the human female body more sensitive to abnormal foetuses.

Dr Carr was one of the first research workers to suggest that spontaneous abortion might be linked with abnormalities in the chromosomes, the tiny rod-shaped particles in the cells which carry genetic information. He has studied fifty-four women who had spontaneous abortions after taking oral contraceptives, and he compared them with a group of 227 women who had also had such abortions but never taken the pill. In the pill-using group the aborted foetuses had a higher ratio of a gross chromosome defect known as triploidy, in which there are not two but three sets of chromosomes.

This could have been the end-result of the pill's interference with the normal balance of hormones in the woman's body. The disequilibrium brought about by chronic dosage with synthetic steroids could have held up the egg's passage from the ovary and its fertilization by the husband's sperm – a train of events known to predispose to triploidy.

Similar results came from an investigation undertaken by a US Army Air Force physician, Colonel William F. Petersen, who spoke at a meeting of the American College of Obstetricians and Gynaecologists in San Diego in late 1968. There was no reason for concern, he said, about either increased or decreased fertility resulting from the pill. But the chances of abortion apparently went up if conception took place within a month after discontinuing oral contraceptives. He had studied 1,141 women who had come under his care at Andrews Air Force Base, Washington DC, during an eight-and-a-half-month period. Well over four hundred of them had taken one or other brand of contraceptive pill, but Petersen considered the numbers too small for valid conclusions. Even so, there was a significantly higher abortion rate among the women who had taken the pill for two years or more and had conceived within a month of discontinuing pill-use. Petersen commented on 'the surprising and disturbing finding' that there was a higher incidence of abortion, premature birth, and birth abnormalities in the women who conceived in the first month after stopping the pill, as against those who conceived later than that. The overall incidence of abortion was essentially the same among the pill-users and the non-pill-users – 9·2 per cent in those who had taken it, 8·6 per cent in those who had not. The chief risk seemed to be run by those mothers whose pregnancies started promptly after they left off taking the pill, and it would be a good idea, Petersen cautioned, to warn any women who wanted to have a baby after using oral contraceptives to avoid conception for the first month.

Though the series was small, the data, he said, 'clearly pinpoint the urgent need for immediate study in this important area'. Many factors remained to be evaluated before the pill could be definitely implicated in his findings.

Laboratory evidence to support the suspicion that the pill is to blame has come from an American surgeon-biochemist working in London, Professor Peter Beaconsfield. At the Royal Free Hospital in 1968, he and Dr Jean Ginsburg performed some experiments with female rats who had been given high doses of progestogen. They left out the oestrogen on the grounds that it had been incriminated as the cause of most of the side-effects and that future oral contraceptives would contain nothing but progestogen. After 120 days on the drug, Beaconsfield's twenty rats were taken off it for fifteen days, then their ovaries were examined. Only in half of them were the ova at a normal stage of development. The others were found to have various kinds of chromosome abnormality indicating arrested development. The researchers also studied the effect on the animal's fertility. Twenty rats which had not been given the drug readily conceived and had the usual eight to ten offspring per litter. But with the rats which had had the progestogen – it was norethynodrel – there were no pregnancies at all for thirty days, after which some did conceive, but only seven of them, and they produced litters of four to six offspring.

*

Reporting their results in the *Lancet* in March 1968, Beaconsfield and Jean Ginsburg had some general comments to make. They wrote that side-effects were bound to occur with any drug. But so far, standards of safety had been balanced against a drug's medical benefits, bearing in mind dosage and the length of time it was taken. Now we faced the prospect of millions of healthy women taking a drug during most of their adult lives for 'non-essential purposes'. Yet we only had limited knowledge of how the drug affected metabolism, what the cumulative effects might be and whether they could be reversed. It would be advisable, they argued, for women taking the pill to give their metabolism a rest at regular intervals, adopting a nine-months-on, three-months-off routine, and reverting to some other form of contraception in the intervals between taking the pill. Meanwhile, new methods of testing ought to be developed to allow more accurate predictions of the long-term effects of drugs intended for continuous dosage.

This *Lancet* report drew a quick reaction from the then Deputy Director of the Family Planning Association, Dr Hilary Hill, and the Chairman of the Council for the Investigation of Fertility Control (CIFC), the endocrinologist Dr Peter Bishop. If you want to study the effect of a drug on people, you should test it on people not rats, they said. Also the doses given to the rats at the Royal Free Hospital were disproportionately high and the drug used, norethynodrel, was not being recommended for use as a progestogen-only contraceptive. As a counterblast to Beaconsfield's twenty rats, they cited a series of sixty-three fertile women from CIFC records who had taken the pill for various periods and then stopped to have babies. All but two of these had conceived (the two who had not were still trying) and the number of miscarriages was lower than the generally accepted number. None of the babies was abnormal. Sixty-three patients was not many, they admitted, but at least it was more than Professor Beaconsfield's rats.

Their letter ended: 'So Professor Beaconsfield and Dr Ginsburg have not studied the same species about which they are issuing disturbing warnings; they have given a progestogen for very long periods of time in high and possibly toxic doses to only twenty rats, whereas it is given either in very small doses continuously or in somewhat larger doses intermittently to women; and they have not used the same progestogen which is given for continuous administration in women' – that is chlormadinone, the progestogen in the 'mini-pill', then under clinical evaluation.

But the two Royal Free workers claimed in reply that the doses given to the rats were in fact far below the toxic level and were consistent with their experimental design. And whatever the results in the sixty-three women from CIFC records, other people who had studied the pill's effects on fertility had come up with less reassuring conclusions.

So, not for the first time, convincing arguments were paraded by either side in support of their point of view. And as with all the reactions, one is left with a series of unanswered questions and a nagging sense of unease, shared as we have seen by many doctors.

It is true that most of the adverse reactions to the pill have so far proved to be reversible: they can usually be put right by the simple expedient of not taking the pill any more. It is also true that in most cases only a few women are affected, or have been so far.

But the doctor who says the adverse reactions are not proven, or so rare as to be negligible, is really asking his patients to trust him beyond the point that is customary in the doctor-patient relationship. Like his patients, he can only wait and see.

# 6. Tiers of Testing

'I am sure that I am not the only physician who is concerned by the literature accumulating on the untoward and often conflicting as yet unknown, effects of long-term pill administration. . . . What is the type of testing for drugs taken in the long-term . . .? Has it been spelt out anywhere and have I missed it? If new testing is required, whose responsibility is it to see that it is done? And in which way can this help to improve the present pill?' –

Dr R. Grenville-Mathers, writing to the *British Medical Journal*, 1968

'In the view of the Dunlop Committee and the large majority of the medical profession, women should be told of such risks as are known or hinted at in contraceptive pills and then allowed to make up their own mind. This, after all, is what emancipation is all about' –

Ann Shearer, *The Guardian*, 1968

Should the pill be banned? The drug safety authorities, on whom the decision rests, evidently do not think so. If the hazards had in their opinion reached the point where wholesale prohibition were called for, the appropriate moves would have been made. When I asked the man who was then (in May 1969) US Commissioner of Food and Drugs, Dr Herbert Ley, what it would take for the pill to be totally withdrawn from prescription in America, he made it clear in the course of a diplomatic reply that it would take much more severe, widespread and unexpected effects than anything reported so far before this decision were contemplated.

Epidemic cancer, the disturbing possibility raised by Dr Roy Hertz's argument, would do it. So would a swift increase in deaths from atherosclerosis. So, probably, would a widespread outbreak of any of the conditions already discussed. As the reports of increased risk pile up, one can foresee, if not an outright ban, an accelerating drift away from 'classical' pill contraception – and, if they are available, a move towards better

and safer types of pill. It is likely to develop into a race between the researchers looking for evidence of risks with the
present pill, and the researchers looking for new pills with no
risks at all.

But perhaps the question is not, should we ban the pill, but
could it be banned? Some five per cent of pill prescriptions are,
ostensibly at least, not for contraceptive purposes but for menstrual disorders. In these cases the pill is not necessarily taken
for long periods and involves a slight risk only. If the pill were
allowed to stay for the treatment of these disorders, one could
also imagine a situation where doctors who remained unimpressed by the evidence of adverse effects, a stubborn rearguard, would go on prescribing the drugs for 'gynaecological
reasons' as is now done in Roman-Catholic countries: a kind of
black market in oral contraceptives.

Nor would the move to ban the pill carry as much weight in
deprived and over-populated countries, where the risks entailed
in pregnancy and childbirth are high enough to cancel out a
risk considerably higher than would be tolerated in the West.

Successive announcements in the winter months of 1969–70
did amount to a piecemeal ban of sorts on some oral contraceptives in some places. They also narrowed down the range of
contraceptive pills women can take without going against the
opinion of one or other of the drug testing bodies in Britain or
the USA. First the high-oestrogen pills were the subject of a
warning by the Drug Safety Committee in Britain (though not
by the FDA). Then progestogen-only pills were withdrawn by
their makers in America, where the FDA had not licensed them
– though the British Drug Safety Committee already had. This
confusing situation demonstrates that the analogous bodies in
Britain and America are not always in step, although they say
they keep in close touch with each other. These authorities bear
the brunt of responsibility in protecting the consumer but, as
recent events prove, they are, inevitably, far from being infallible.

The whole question of drug safety and the efficiency of testing procedures – for drugs new and old – has grown more and
more complex with the increasing ingenuity of the pharma-

ceutical chemists. It is not made any easier by the large number of new drugs put forward every year by the companies for official approval. As many as 820 new submissions were made to the British Drug Safety Committee in 1969: most of these (some ninety per cent) were not exactly new, but reformulations of existing drugs. This does not exempt the committee's officials from painstaking review of the data supplied, to eliminate as far as possible the risk of adverse effects.

In America the position is much the same. The total number of new applications is around seven hundred to eight hundred a year, I was told at the FDA's Washington office. Again a large proportion of these are reformulations of drugs already on the market.

The testing procedure for new oral contraceptive pills laid down by the FDA is more rigorous than for other drugs. The rules were stiffened after a new oral contraceptive, undergoing clinical trials in 1966, was found to produce abnormalities in the breasts of women taking part. The trial was summarily terminated and the product withdrawn. The minimum requirement now is a one-year study of the drug's toxicity in rodents and dogs before there is any initial clinical trial. This trial usually consists of a three-month study with women subjects. The FDA also recommends that, concurrently, there should be a study of the drug's chronic effects in monkeys. The three month clinical trial with women is only a preliminary, and eventually the drug would have to go successfully through large-scale trials lasting a year or more before being passed for general prescription. But before this, the FDA insists on the manufacturers embarking on long-term tests with animals – seven years with dogs, and ten years with monkeys. If the manufacturers put forward an application to market a product, they have to submit the results of at least two years' testing on dogs, rats and monkeys.

Animal tests consist of very much more than just giving the drug to the animals and waiting to see if they become ill or die. The routine of testing includes deliberate overdosage, tests of the drug's effects on the foetus and tests of its hormonal activity.

The clinical trials themselves are directed by a private

research worker or a research organization with access to the appropriate type of patient, and they are carried out according to a protocol devised or approved by the FDA. Initial clinical trials are used to assess the product's ability to inhibit ovulation; as we have seen, these are based on analyses of urine, vaginal smear, specimens of tissues in the womb and sometimes a minor surgical operation to inspect the ovaries. If the results are acceptable the drug is put to trial as a contraceptive, a variety of doses and combination of doses being used.

In Britain, the Drug Safety Committee's requirements are more flexible. The Committee asks for comprehensive information about a drug's pharmacology and also the results of clinical trials with a large number of patient-cycles. It does lay down rigorous rules for screening possible cancerous effects.

The criteria on which approval for new contraceptive pills is based have become more stringent over the years, partly because of greater scepticism towards drugs in general. When the first oral contraceptives were introduced they were not required to go through this complicated routine; but the FDA has ruled that all contraceptive pills licensed before 1966 must be submitted to prolonged toxicity tests on animals, and the results reported to Washington.

Some would argue that even this is not enough. One man who takes this view is Professor Peter Beaconsfield, of the Royal Free Hospital in London, whose experiments involving the administration of large doses of progestogen to rats have already been mentioned. Beaconsfield maintains that by and large the testing routines used for the pill are appropriate to a different kind of drug, the kind taken for purely medicinal purposes, and designed for use over relatively short periods when side-effects matter less. The pill is the first of what could be a long series of 'social' drugs, intended not for the sick but the healthy, and meant to be taken for years on end – such as contraceptive pills for men, or pills for greying hair. But Beaconsfield believes that most of the research now going on into the pill's safety is inadequate for the purpose, because it is based on statistical, epidemiological studies: it is 'wrongly orientated', he says. More and more women are taking the pill, yet medicine can apparently suggest no way of finding out what the long-term effects might be, except to wait and see what comes out of the statistics.

Beaconsfield's solution is for what he calls a 'two-tier' testing system. The first tier comprises the kind of tests applied at present for standard medicinal drugs. The second tier should be, he says, a systematic study of the pill's effects on detailed cell function and structure. The object would be to ensure that the drug's effects on the vital organs are within normal limits and do not cause any serious change in the cell's architecture; that any changes caused should not be cumulative and should be capable of being reversed when the drug is discontinued; and that there should be no effects on the cell's capacity to reproduce itself.

He further argues that the techniques for doing this already exist, and that the experimental material could be either animal or human tissues taken soon after death. About one-third of all deaths in urban society are caused by accidents, he says, and there must be a proportion of these who were women who had been on the pill for some time. 'It should not be beyond the powers of our organizational abilities,' he wrote recently, 'to make arrangements with coroners that tissue samples be available from such cases for research studies.' In his experience, he added, coroners were quite ready to cooperate.

In contributions to medical journals Beaconsfield has summed up his view of the problem in the phrase 'Side-effects are end-effects'. 'This concept is I think the only thing that I have contributed to the argument,' he said to me urbanely. 'After all, my results are so small in depth and scope. But what I mean is this. Some women for example who take the pill become depressed. Some slow down generally and behave like pregnant ladies, they are much more flaccid, it takes them twenty minutes to write a letter instead of ten, and so on. The slowing down is the result of a number of processes, things happening to the brain, to the hormone balance, the general biochemical constituents in the body. It is the metabolism which has slowed down. Everything has changed, but the clinical symptom of slowness is the end-effect of a number of biochemical and biophysical events. Any side-effect in medicine is the end-effect of a long biochemical process, and to understand it you have to go back to the start of the process and see what is happening.'

Not everyone would agree that the task of pinpointing the biochemical mischief caused by the pill can be done as simply as Beaconsfield suggests. But assuming it can, the next question is, who is to carry out the testing? When I put this to Beaconsfield, during our talk in a modest prefabricated building in the Royal Free's branch in the Liverpool Road, he said:

Of course, you can't expect a clinical department like this to take it on, you require a set-up which is infinitely more specialized than we are.

I have suggested a meeting should be called publicly, to decide what to look for, and how to look for it. A small meeting, run essentially by clinicians, about twenty or twenty-four people, with good knowledge of the basic sciences and ready to ask for specialist opinion. That was my suggestion. Everybody said, Beaconsfield, you're nuts. According to them, I'd never find that many cooperative, unbiased experts, all free of vested interests.

When it was first put forward over a year ago, Beaconsfield's proposal for a two-tier testing system was supported by Lady Summerskill, who made it the basis for renewing her demand that the pill should be withdrawn completely. But in general it appears to have been ignored.

Certainly neither the FDA nor the Drug Safety Committee, even if they wished to, could themselves undertake any testing procedures. Neither body has the facilities to test drugs, but has to rely on information submitted to them by drug companies, or which comes their way from medical journal reports, or is volunteered by research groups or reported by individual doctors. They have it in their power to suggest research projects, and in the case of the risks of thrombo-embolism associated with the pill, both the Drug Safety Committee and the FDA did just that. They are, and have often been called, watch-dog organizations. If any significant evidence should be uncovered linking the pill, or any drug, with some unsuspected reaction, it is their duty to raise the alarm – or rather, as they would prefer, to put the matter right *without* causing alarm among the innocent consumers.

When the pill was first launched, the problem of adverse reactions to drugs was taken less seriously. The FDA was in existence, for the Food and Drugs Act on which its work was originally based was passed in 1906; but its standards were not as strict as they have later become and there was no Drug Safety Committee in Britain at all. That committee, brought into being, as we have seen, after the thalidomide disaster, began work in 1964, and at least has the advantage of having been created to do a specific and fairly well defined task. This is one reason why this committee, the Dunlop, or Scowen Committee (Sir Derrick Dunlop was its first Chairman; he resigned in 1969 to become first Director of the Medicines Commission and he was succeeded by Professor Eric Scowen) has escaped most of the criticisms which have stormed around the FDA.

Whichever way one looks at it, running any such body as a drug-licensing committee in a medically sophisticated country must be regarded as one of the most stressful jobs in medicine. This is especially so in America, where the FDA is part of a politically sensitive unit of government, the Department of Health, Education and Welfare. The FDA Commissioner is responsible before the legislature for the actions of his agency and at the mercy of political pressure. And unlike the Scowen Committee, which goes about its work with little public fuss, the FDA has to conduct its business in front of the entire news-reading, television-watching public. Often held up in Britain as the prototype of an efficient, powerful drug-monitoring organization ('the agency that banned thalidomide'), the FDA in its own country is used to being slated for its bureaucratic delays and general toothlessness in protecting the safety of the consumer.

It is not easy to keep pace with the steady stream of what the drug industry likes to think of as, by and large, significant new advances in pharmaceutical chemistry. Both the FDA and the Scowen Committee have to put up with a continuous drone of criticism from the drug firms for their alleged procrastination in dealing with new applications. In the British case, the complaints seem undeserved, since the delay in handling applications is trifling compared with the situation in Washington. In the course of a lengthy comparison of the British and American systems published in 1967, Dr Joseph D. Cooper, Professor of Government at Howard University, Washington DC, found little good to say about the FDA and commented unfavourably on the contrast between Britain's 'lean and spare' drug safety apparatus and the unwieldy system developed over the years in the USA. He reported that the review of new drug applications in Britain took an average of three months for major submissions and from one to two weeks for minor ones. Sometimes, he found to his evident amazement, decisions on minor matters went out by return post. A determined effort, he found, was made to reach decisions as expeditiously as possible 'in order not to deny therapeutic benefit to the public'. He went on: 'The American story, in sharp contrast, is characterized by delay which seems to serve little purpose other than to assure bureaucratic safety. Processing periods of two and three years are not uncommon.'

According to some critics, the American decision not to allow thalidomide drugs to be prescribed, thus escaping the disastrous consequences of the drug in Europe, only happened because the FDA had the application buried in its pending file. By the time it surfaced, the drug's effects on the foetus were already known. If this is true, one can only conclude that bureaucracy sometimes pays.

The FDA's policy of delay – whether it is deliberate or not – also paid off in the case of the 'mini-pill' 'Normenon'. Its use as a low-dose, continuous contraceptive pill containing no oestrogen was first proposed in the mid-sixties. It had large-scale trials in America and Mexico, and in 1969 it was approved by the British Drug Safety Committee, who were probably impressed by the evidence assembled by British doctors showing that 'Normenon' allowed blood-clotting tendencies caused by the classical pill to return to normal. But in spite of restiveness among some of the executives at Syntex in Palo Alto, the FDA did not give final approval. Their hesitation was dramatically justified, it seemed, when in January 1970 Syntex themselves withrew 'Normenon'.

One of the more recent outcries impugning the FDA's efficiency resulted from the exposure of certain irregularities in the system for screening new drugs. It shows how, despite the fine mesh of the filtering process, the system can go wrong. Trials of a process for removing plasma from donor's blood and reinjecting it had been placed in the hands of a private testing corporation which had used it on 376 Alabama convicts, three of whom had died after an outbreak of hepatitis which was found to be due to a 'breakdown' in precautions against sepsis. A prison doctor concerned with the trial was also, it emerged, an associate of the testing corporation. The Alabama Medical Association conducted its own inquiry into what had happened, and described the prison doctor's work, and that of the corporation's medical chief, as 'bluntly, unacceptable' and 'distinctly unsatisfactory'. The trial had been run, the Association considered, without adequate medical supervision or enough trained staff, and with insufficient interest in the prisoners as patients. Prisoners had been pressured into signing consent forms for participation in the trial and those who had been taken ill during it had not had satisfactory medical treatment.

The disclosures were followed shortly afterwards by an announcement from Dr Herbert Ley, then Federal Drugs Commissioner, that immediate steps would be taken to tighten up supervision of the estimated fifteen thousand individuals eligible to conduct testing.

Pressure on the FDA caused by, among other things, new drug applications, comes to the surface most often in the form of complaints about lack of staff and lack of money. Yet compared with the secretariat of a couple of dozen working for the British Drug Safety Committee, the FDA's staff is multitudinous. 'One must soon ask,' Professor Cooper sourly observed, 'whether more people now make their living by talking about drug safety than are in near peril from drugs.'

The FDA as a whole uses a staff of over four thousand and the Bureau of Medicine, which handles the new drug applications, employs some six hundred of them; but the FDA is commonly described as hampered by chronic shortages of personnel and cash. Of the two deficiencies, shortage of the right people was regarded by the FDA officials I spoke to as the harder to remedy. 'We are not under any illusion that money alone would do it,' said Dr Harvey Minchew, then head of the Bureau. Dr Minchew, who was about to leave the FDA to go to Johns Hopkins University, added, 'After all, who wants to spend his time here reviewing someone else's data?'

An internal report on the FDA's activities, from the FDA itself and produced in 1969, described it as 'currently not equipped to cope with the challenge' it faced as the country's main agency for the protection of the consumer. The reasons were identified, once again, as insufficient money and staff – and, in addition, insufficient legal authority.

The departure of Dr Herbert Ley at the end of 1969, and his replacement as Commissioner by Dr Charles C. Edwards, were the start of a reshuffle within the FDA, followed by more public self-criticism, this time on the part of Dr Edwards. Describing the new reforms he had introduced, he indicated to a congressional subcommittee that his scrutiny of FDA affairs had been a disturbing experience. 'The decision-making environment was disorderly,' he said, 'professional talent was stifled, poorly directed, and unmotivated. Planning was shockingly myopic.'

When it comes to monitoring adverse reactions to drugs, FDA spokesmen point out, they still have no authority to compel doctors to report to them any cases they come across of an untoward side-effect from the contraceptive pill or any other drug prescribed.

In this respect the FDA is like the Scowan Committee, which also has no legal authority to require doctors to send in their reports. But unlike the FDA, it does not have the power to withdraw a drug. It can only recommend doctors not to prescribe it, although a recommendation to that effect from such an authoritative body would have the same force as an outright ban.

In spite of everything, however, serious mishaps with drug safety are rare. Nothing approaching the scale of the thalidomide disaster has happened since that traumatic event, and if the thalidomide experience has made the drug safety authorities over-cautious, this is how the consumers would undoubtedly prefer it. Nevertheless, one of the crucial questions is how efficient the monitoring system is for a drug which has passed the initial safety precautions and reached the market.

To a considerable extent, both bodies are in the hands of the doctors who prescribe. The early warning system used by the Drug Safety Committee relies on the cooperation, and the conscience, of individual doctors. The system's main equipment consists of the 'yellow cards': reply-paid cards of which every doctor (and dentist) has in theory his own supply, and which he is expected to fill in and return to the Committee's offices in London with details of the drug used, the patient it was used on and how long for, what other drugs were being taken – and the adverse reaction suspected. An adverse reaction is defined as one which is noxious, unintended, and occurring with doses normally used in treatment.

Between three and four thousand yellow cards are returned every year, about three-quarters of them from family doctors and the rest from doctors in hospitals. But periodically, the Committee complains through its officials of the small number of cards returned, though the quality of the reports received have been described by Dr Dennis Cahal, formerly the Committee's Medical Assessor, as 'remarkably good'. As an illustration of the laxity of doctors, the Committee points to its investigations into thrombo-embolism and the pill. When they checked back to find how many of the known deaths from thrombo-embolism among women using the pill had actually been reported to the Committee, they were shocked to discover that doctors had only notified them of fifteen per cent of the cases. This was despite the fact that on several occasions the link between the pill and clotting diseases had been the subject of massive publicity in the popular as well as the medical press. 'If under-reporting has occurred to such an extent on a topic so full of emotion and so widely publicized as oral contraceptives,' Cahal asked recently, 'to what extent has it occurred on topics less charged with drama?'

In the United States, drug safety officials are equally worried over the problem. So sketchily had doctors reported deaths from clotting episodes in America in 1965 that the returns on this subject were declared 'virtually useless' in the FDA's 1966 report on the pill. FDA officials say that one of the difficulties they have to face is lack of the direct contact with the individual doctor which the Scowen Committee can claim. 'What we do not have,' said Dr Minchew, 'is any system for feed-in of data from the practitioner. We are interested in this. But nothing is operational.' Matters are easier, I was told, where there is a National Health Service and a 'proper channel of communication' between doctor and the executive arm of government. 'In this country,' Commissioner Herbert Ley tactfully remarked, 'doctors have somewhat of a negative bias towards communication with the government rather than their own Association.' The contrast is probably not as stark as Dr Ley believed: but it is true that the American system for monitoring adverse reactions is not as comprehensive as the one in Britain. It is understood that any doctor with something to report will contact not the FDA but the firm which manufactured the drug in question. They in turn notify the FDA. The system no doubt springs as much from mistrust of federal surveillance as from respect for the sturdy independence of American business. The manufacturers themselves are required to pass on information to Washington at three-monthly intervals during the first year of a product's life, half-yearly in the second year and annually thereafter. If anything dramatic should happen in the way of side-effect, the companies have to report the fact within fifteen working days of it coming to their notice.

Besides this, the FDA has contracts with fifty-two hospitals throughout the United States (it used to be eighty but the number was cut in 1969 because of 'budgetary restrictions') under which the hospitals make a return of adverse reactions once a month. And there are also more specific contracts with a small number of research centres covering the 'methodology' of monitoring reactions.

The FDA doctors admit that they are concerned over the inadequacy of this system, but say they can point to occasions when it has worked well in swiftly removing a drug from prescription when untoward effects occur. Slow to license, quick to ban : if this is the policy it is certainly better than the other way round. One case instanced by the FDA was a drug for the control of nausea and dizziness which was withdrawn six months after its introduction, having been found to cause visual and auditory hallucinations in a small number of patients. The first warning the FDA received came from the manufacturers themselves – who willingly withdrew the product.

But though it is usual to pay polite tribute to the cooperation of the industry, in the interests of better relations all round, not every company is as ready or as able to help as the makers of that particular drug. It is not necessarily bull-headedness so much as sloppy organization. The drug industry's grumbles about the FDA's inefficiency sound odd when one considers the results of the special inquiry carried out for the FDA in 1966 by Dr Schuyler D. Kohl, of King's County Medical Centre, who was asked to look into the way pill-manufacturing firms kept their records and conducted their investigations of adverse reactions. Almost without exception, Dr Kohl acknowledged, the people responsible for monitoring drug safety among the seven firms making oral contraceptives were 'competent and interested in their work'. But not all the firms were above reproach. Although Dr Kohl discreetly refrained from identifying which was which, the medical departments of the manufacturers were, he said, quite variable. 'Some are very sophisticated in approach and personnel and one occupies a "basement office" and is quite restricted in personnel and outlook.' Each manufacturer had a number of 'investigational patients' who had been under observation for a known period of time: sometimes there were as many as twenty thousand patients in a firm's series. The records of adverse reactions, he found, were in general quite complete, but some were 'skimpy' and there was a lot of variation in the rigorousness with which a patient was followed up. And there was no uniform way of recording all the information collected, so that any attempt to put it all together into a coherent series would have been somewhat difficult.

Some of the statistical analysis done in the drug firms Dr Kohl characterized as 'naïve', and it certainly seems that there were some glaring omissions. An important one, for instance, was the lack of follow-up of the few patients who became pregnant while they were taking the pill. Almost without exception there was a dearth of information on the outcome of their pregnancies, which Kohl mildly said 'might be of importance in both medical and epidemiological areas of interest'.

Detailed ways in which the whole situation could be improved included some suggestions addressed to the FDA, who were advised to lay down clearer guidelines to the industry on exactly what they wanted reported to them and generally to establish better communications with the drug firms. Among the recommendations of the FDA's Committee on Obstetrics and Gynaecology, in the first report on the pill, it was said that there was every evidence that the drug firms were willing and anxious to cooperate with the FDA and with each other 'to achieve more efficient surveillance and more meaningful data.' A conference was suggested by the Committee, at which the FDA and the respective drug firms could discuss uniformity and increased efficiency in reporting. Three years later, when the FDA's second report on the pill came out, that conference had still not been held.

Whatever arrangements are made for collecting, processing and reporting large quantities of statistics on the pill's unwanted effects, the raw material for statistics, without which any arrangement is bound to collapse, comes from the experience and observations of doctors. This is the source of the data the drug safety authorities want for early warning purposes and there is no substitute for it. In America, the FDA Committee noted, the system relied on 'either the cooperation of physicians or the haphazard filtering of rumours to detail men' – the travelling representatives of the drug companies whose job is to 'detail' (i.e. inform) doctors about the benefits of their firms' products. The Committee added despondently: 'The latter route is patently unreliable and the former not much better.'

In fact the starting point for either route remains the same: the prescribing doctor. Laziness, lack of interest, too much work to do – these are some of the reasons why doctors do not report the adverse reactions they see. In America, some doctors do not report because they dislike handing over to a commercial firm confidential information about their patients. Another powerful deterrent, in America at least, is fear of legal action. Reporting a death, or even a non-fatal side-effect, from a drug he has prescribed might be regarded as a tacit admission by the doctor that he was to blame. There were believed to be in 1970 over a hundred lawsuits pending in the USA against pill-manufacturing firms or doctors, moved by aggrieved patients or, in some tragic cases, their widowed husbands. The undoubted increase in the number of actions brought against doctors is to some extent a result of the 'litigation fever' which can often be satisfied by suing practitioners of so inexact a science as medicine. To a lesser extent, the same is true in Britain, where the Medical Defence Union – the largest of the medical protection societies – has consistently reported year by year increases in the amount of money handed over on its 63,000 members' behalf in indemnity payments, legal charges and other disbursements. 'Doctors,' commented an eminent New York gynaecologist, 'are a high risk profession. Why, my malpractice insurance has gone up in twelve years from thirty to a thousand dollars a year.' He was luckier than he knew, to judge from a report in 1969 that in California it was 'not unusual' for surgeons to pay between $7,500 and $12,000 a year (£3,100 to £5,000) in insurance premiums to cover themselves against the risk of malpractice suits. At least in Britain the doctor has the medical protection societies to act for him, and in return for a peppercorn subscription: six guineas a year.

Expecting a doctor to report side-effects for the pill presupposes that the doctor knows they have occurred. But often the assumption is without foundation. FDA official Dr John J. Schrogie wrote in June 1969: 'It is no exaggeration to say that these relatively inexpensive drugs have often been dispensed without the traditional safeguards and continuing valuation of patients that ordinarily are practised in chronic drug therapy. Perhaps because of this less intensive review, it has taken much longer for us to clearly appreciate the multiple biological effects of the oral contraceptives. Yet, some of these effects were in fact readily predictable on the basis of available information.'

'There's no doubt at all,' said one London GP, 'that some doctors haven't the vaguest idea what happens to their patients who take the pill for the simple reason that once they've given the prescription they never see them. The patients are jolly lucky if they get any sort of examination, too. You want the pill, dear? Right you are, out comes the prescription pad and hey presto, a year's supply of the first one he thinks of.' The same doctor suggested: 'If you want an idea of the kind of slap-happy prescribing that goes on, for the pill or anything else, you want to have a word with one or two chemists! Get them to tell you about the women who come in with the same old dog-eared repeat prescription, every so often, for their supply of contraceptive pills.'

In a survey of nearly two thousand general practitioners carried out in 1968 by the Institute of Community Studies, in London, the doctors who prescribed the pill (the great majority of the sample) were asked the length of time for which the prescriptions were given. Nearly three-quarters of them gave a prescription for three months, or less, to begin with and nearly a third gave only one month's supply. But one in four of the doctors straightaway gave out prescriptions for 'at least a year'. A postal questionnaire conducted by Syntex in Britain in 1968 showed that twenty-seven per cent of GPs did not re-examine their pill-taking patients for two years or more (with consultants the figure was two per cent). And when *The Sun* a few months later asked for readers' experiences with the pill, the shoals of correspondence on every imaginable aspect of the subject included some disturbing evidence of the haphazard way the pill was being prescribed. 'Letter after letter,' wrote the paper's Woman's Editor, 'tells of doctors writing prescriptions without even cursory questioning, let alone examination. One mother of four recounts how she was put on the pill without a blood pressure test although she had already had a thrombosis.'

That this kind of misuse of drugs goes on is common knowledge among doctors – and chemists – and, to a less extent, patients. Probably only a minority of doctors are guilty: no one

has ever had the temerity to publish any investigation which
would throw light on the matter.

Women who attend family planning clinics for their contraceptive pill (well over 400,000 in Britain, out of more than
1,800,000 taking the pill) are at least promised the right
amount of medical surveillance. They will be screened for
breast and cervical cancer, have their blood pressure taken and
also a thorough medical history. They will be seen again six
weeks after they have started on the pill, then every six months.
All this – plus the opportunity, if they want it, to talk over any
sex problems they may have, and the chance, as Dr Hilary Hill,
formerly Deputy Director (Medical) of the Family Planning Association, put it, 'to weep on somebody's shoulder'.

Of course, they will have to pay for their supply of pills (26p
to 46p, depending on brand, for a month's supply) and a clinic
charge of £3.00 for the first year and £2.00 for every subsequent
year. Oddly, the woman who gets contraceptive pills through her
family doctor may also have to pay: not only the over-the-
counter cost at the pharmacy (around 45p. for a month's
supply), she will also have to pay her doctor, unless he is prepared to waive the charge because of medical or social necessity. Oddly, because there is no other prescribing act performed
by National Health Service doctors for which they are able to
make a charge. Fears that general practitioners might be
'swamped' by importunate demands for free contraceptives led
the British Medical Association, when the pill was first introduced, to insist on an appropriate charge being made. In BMA
discussions at the time, it was clear that many general practitioners considered that there was something undignified and
even a little unsavoury about being expected to dole out contraceptives on the National Health. Thus, family doctors are
advised by the BMA to charge 70p in return for an oral contraceptive prescription valid for six months, while prescriptions for
every other drug in the pharmacopoeia cost nothing – another
way in which the pill is unique.

If a woman is getting the pill from a clinic, the clinic notifies
her family doctor, and indeed gives him the opportunity to say
whether he knows of any medical reason against her having it.

Thus, in theory at least, every general practitioner with a patient taking oral contraceptives is in command of the situation. If one of those patients becomes ill, he should remember or have a note of the fact, that she is on the pill, and not only bear this in mind if he has to prescribe some other drug, but be ready to ask himself whether the pill could have anything to do with her illness. All this is more easily said than done: letters get lost, records are not consulted in time, the doctor might simply forget. But the individual doctor is the vital link in the chain of responsibility for any early warning system. And on the drug safety authorities' own admission, that link is also one of the weakest.

What of the patients themselves? 'Every woman should be free to make up her own mind,' said one doctor I spoke to, 'with the judicious guidance of her own doctor. She must know the hazards of the pill, where they exist, and be helped to balance those hazards against others, some of which perhaps she takes for granted.' It sounds admirable and it is a point of view to which most doctors would subscribe: but it is impossible in all but a few cases to achieve this satisfactory state of balance. In Washington at the beginning of 1970 a series of Congressional hearings was held to find out whether women were told enough about the dangers of the pill. One result was a new FDA ruling that supplies of oral contraceptives sold in the US should include a leaflet warning of possible hazards. In fact, a warning of a kind had been included for a long time by manufacturers – but the pharmacist always took it out. All the American woman has had to read in the past has been a cheery leaflet explaining such things as how to get the tablets out of the foil, and, perhaps, some information on minor side-effects. There was also a caution that 'any unusual changes in health' should be reported to the doctor. Not that the longer warning would have been especially enlightening to anyone but a doctor. It mentioned various types of clotting disease and a host of other conditions from itching to hirsutism – but in the style of a medical journal. The new leaflet is to be in simple language. (The arguments over its wording will be described later.) Meanwhile in Britain there is no ruling from the Drug Safety Com-

mittee on package information. A simple leaflet goes with the
pills which warns of minor side-effects and suggests a visit to
the doctor if the woman notices anything unusual.

As for other sources of information, there are always the
newspapers. But journalists who report the hazards of the pill
are used to accusations of 'press sensationalism' and 'scare reporting': usually it is a coroner who has supplied the sensation
– one thinks of the coroner who publicly condemned the pill as
'this dangerous medicament'. The press does make, however,
a useful scapegoat for the disagreements within the medical
profession over whether the pill is safe. At the beginning of
1970 the British Council's *Medical Bulletin* produced a special
issue on fertility control, one of the contributors to which cited
the statement that the extra deaths each year attributable to the
pill were five out of every 800,000 women, while during the
same period thirty-five women in every 800,000 would have
been killed in road accidents. Another contribution, from Professor Sir Richard Doll and Dr Martin Vessey, noted that
nobody knew how often events reported as adverse reactions to
the pill occurred among the general population who were not
taking it. Introducing the issue, Sir Alan Parkes had this to say:
'Unfortunately, it is probably too much to hope that even
papers such as these will undo the harm done by alarmist headlines in the national press, for which one woman whose death
could possibly be attributed to oral contraception has naturally
greater news value than a thousand women who are healthy
and happy using it.'

Yet if women are to know about the hazards of the pill,
established or suspected, if they are to make the sort of informed decision doctors say they expect, the bad news has to
be reported. Women have the right to know the worst. They,
after all, are the consumers – and possibly, the victims.

# 7 A Pill for The People

*'The price of the "pill" is too much to find out of their grants, complain girl students at Canterbury University. They want a half-penny off the retail price – 5d each ... As one girl remarked: "Discounts help us meet the cost of living. It seems stupid that there should be this sort of discrimination against the 'pill'".'* –

Medical News, 1967

*'What a dismal treadmill is love on the pill!'* –

Malcolm Muggeridge, 1968

While the medical argument over safety and side-effects continues, it does so largely over the heads of the eighteen million or more women all over the world who go on taking the pill – most of them without the slightest overt sign of illness or incapacity or any special concern about what the long-term side-effects might be. They may have moments of anxiety now and again, and especially when the debate inside medicine explodes into the press or on television. Bafflement and worry is one reaction: who are the women to believe? Consult your doctor, they are told. But the doctor may not know any more than he has read in the papers, and he is probably one of the majority of doctors who consider the risks too small to worry about – less than pregnancy, less than smoking, less than driving a car. There are other forms of contraception, but the pill is so certain – and so convenient.

Some women are scared off the pill. Some carry on, but with a little more unease than before. Some just shrug it off. Gradually the scare is forgotten: down go the pills as usual, and upward climbs the graph of world-wide pill consumption.

This is what seems to have followed the British Drug Safety Committee's announcement in December 1969 about pills with a high oestrogen content. Reports of adverse reactions had shown that clotting disease was occurring more often in women taking high-oestrogen pills. The Committee was therefore recommending, said the Chairman Professor Eric Scowen, that pills containing the smaller doses of oestrogen should normally be prescribed.

Publication of this information in the national press before it reached the medical journals enraged a good many doctors, and the *British Medical Journal*'s correspondence pages were filled with indignant letters protesting at the Committee's 'rude' and 'maladroit' handling of the affair. At least, however, it ensured that the news went swiftly home to the consumer. But doctors coping with a flu epidemic and the usual ills of winter were suddenly deluged with requests for advice about the safety of oral contraceptives and, specifically, the one the caller was actually taking. 'Short of a declaration of war by a foreign power,' wrote Dr Ian MacQueen, Medical Officer of Health for Aberdeen and head of the city's extensive family planning service, 'nothing could have caused greater gloom and chaos.' Conflicting advice had been offered by the Scowen Committee, the Family Planning Association and the medical journals, he wrote angrily in *The Medical Officer:* the only thing they agreed about was that women should not panic.

But the panic was soon over. Nothing had been banned, after all, and women were reassured that the Scowen Committee had not said anything about an *increased* risk: the risk was the same as it had been the day before the announcement and the evidence on which their statement was made had still to be made public. One spokesman for the pill-manufacturing companies said, 'I reckon a lot of women just thought, oh, the hell with it – and went on taking the same pill as before. A lot must have changed to the low-dose variety, but not as many as everybody anticipated.'

A woman doctor at a family planning clinic commented: 'we were inundated with calls when the news broke. But the queer thing was, most of the women said, not "Is the pill I'm on dangerous?" but "I hope this doesn't mean I've got to stop taking the pill". Actually we'd already changed to low-dose oestrogen for nearly all the patients so it didn't make much difference to us.'

It is another demonstration of patients' loyalty to oral contraception. For millions of women who take it and suffer no symptoms worth the name, the pill is still – for the time being – the boon they thought it would be, still the passport to what one user ecstatically described as 'an unsuspected world of good health and sexual wellbeing'. The main point about the pill to most of its consumers is that to all intents and purposes it is the only one hundred per cent reliable contraceptive. From the straightforward point of view of family limitation and never mind the side-effects, the oral contraceptive is the answer to the family planner's dream. Now and again, pregnancies do occur – the Drug Safety Committee has asked doctors to report them, treating such pregnancies, ironically, as though they were like any other unwanted side-effect. But many doctors insist that when a woman on the pill becomes pregnant, it is not the pill that fails, but the pill-user: she forgot to take one or two during the month. Swallow it regularly, according to the instructions, and fear of pregnancy has gone. And with it, in millions of cases, goes any number of inhibitions which spoil enjoyment of sex. Using the pill makes you a different woman, as doctors and patients enthusiastically testify – different in many senses, and not least in distinguishing today's woman from women throughout history, for whom it was never possible to separate completely the pleasurable from the procreative purposes of sex.

The point has not been lost on the manufacturers. FIFTY YEARS OF EMANCIPATION, ran a headline over one of the Eli Lilly company's advertisements for their sequential contraceptive pill: NOW WITH THIS NEW ORAL CONTRACEPTIVE WOMAN'S FREEDOM IS COMPLETE. The picture shows a two-horse dray, *circa* 1913, decorated with suffragette slogans and driven by a militant group of women activists. Not only does woman now have the vote, the text of the advertisement points out, she also has freedom to plan her family as she chooses. Implicit is another freedom: to enjoy sex for its own sake as men have always been able to. 'It was marvellous,' said one

London housewife who took the pill for more than a year. 'You feel free. I mean, I thought to myself, now I can have an affair just like he can and whenever I want one.' The appearance of a few broken veins on her legs and face made her go back, on the clinic's advice, to using a diaphragm, and her freedom was short-lived. But millions of other women possess it still and will go on doing so.

The scientific and social precedents for systemic contraception are firmly established and it is difficult to imagine the clock being put back now. If the pill is here to stay, despite its hazards, society has more convulsions to endure before it is taken for granted. Little by little, men are growing used to a permanent alteration in the balance of sexual power, a shift in the customary roles of men and women. Man the hunter, and woman the shrinking quarry – these prototypes are beginning to recede into legend. 'There is nothing some girls like better,' reported a woman family planning doctor to a Bristol conference of the Royal College of General Practitioners, 'than to dictate to their boy friends not only the method of birth control they wish to use, but also the position adopted in intercourse.' With the pill, contraception is entirely the woman's responsibility : the idea of passive femininity is out of place. A series of surveys carried out among eighteen-year-olds in Leicestershire convinced Dr William Kind, a school medical officer, that because of the pill 'the girls are becoming more emancipated, and the boys are afraid they are going to get emotionally carved up by them'. His conclusion finds a parallel in the opinion of the Chicago psychiatrist who wrote that 'the liberating effect of the pill on the wife evokes all the latent emotional and sexual immaturity in the husband, once he is faced with real demands on his sexuality'. But convinced supporters of female sexual emancipation shed no tears over such a predicament. 'Well hard luck,' was one woman's comment on the psychiatrist's observation. 'It's about time real demands were made on some of these sexually aggressive males – the kind of self-satisfied blowhard who blames his wife's frigidity if their sex lives are no good. If the pill helps to expose that kind of emotional fraud, hooray for the pill.'

The pill's effect on sexual *mores* is one of those huge, vague subjects in which guesswork can be given its head: everyone's speculation has about equal credibility. The remarkable thing is how the pill has worked its way into the fabric of social life in the West, with its own mythology of jokes and tall stories. (The best known, never traced to an authoritative source, told of a teenage girl who stole her mother's contraceptive pills, replacing them – improbably, since they are not at all alike – with aspirins. The payoff, according to one version: mother became pregnant, daughter contracted VD.)

Such is the enthusiasm with which the contraceptive steroids have been taken up that it does not seem the least surprising that a contraceptive pill for dogs has become available ('Ovarid': on vets' prescription only) nor that, according to a rather close-mouthed spokesman for the manufacturers, 'It is reasonable to presume that research is also being done into producing a similar contraceptive for cats.' Why not? After all, an experimental attempt has reputedly been made off the North-American coast to keep down the seagull population – in the interests of aircraft safety – by concealing 350,000 contraceptive pills in herrings, and fish have also been given contraceptive compounds to increase their fertility – off the Isle of Man. They were given the compound for three months, then treatment was stopped, and the fish spawned forthwith. More than once it has been suggested that the pigeon population in cities should be controlled by putting oestrogen into synthetic grit feeding pellets: it would reduce the fertility of mature pigeons, sterilize immature birds – and keep buildings and statues smear-free. Pig-breeders, too, can regulate sows' breeding cycles by drugs which suppress ovulation. And chemical control of ovulation in sheep has been offered to farmers for several years: the whole flock becomes fertile simultaneously, and so lambing is synchronized and the ram only has to pay one visit. Meantime poultry farmers also have been able to take advantage of the new contraceptive techniques, by mixing anti-ovulatory hormones in with the birds' mash. In Scorton, Lancs, the owner of 2,500 turkeys and five hundred geese was able to postpone egg-production among a proportion of his birds until after the months of glut. 'There hasn't been a single slip-up,' he reported complacently. 'Not one egg has been laid by any bird put on the pill.'

Profitable in the short term no doubt, but the people who eat the eggs and bacon at the other end of the production line might like to have a say in the matter, if they only knew. Nobody has yet investigated the long-term effect of eating foods from animals treated in this way : it may well be that the added chemicals would not survive long enough to do any damage. Like so many of the pill's effects, it is an open question, though in this case probably a minor one. Nevertheless it has to be taken together with the discovery a short time ago that minute traces of contraceptive steroids had been discovered in London's water supply. The short-lived scare this discovery caused was probably due as much as anything to the realization – unfamiliar to many – that Londoners were drinking water that had, as it were, been round more than once, for the chemicals had reached the water from the urine of women who were taking the pill. Fears that the male population was being gradually caponized were set at rest by the reassurance from the Ministry of Housing and Local Government that only by drinking three to four pints of water daily for twenty-five years would one swallow the equivalent of one contraceptive pill.

Some of the other social by-products of the pill's arrival have given less cause for disquiet. In New York the National Retail Merchants Association blamed the pill for a twenty per cent drop in sales of maternity wear. In London, lingerie firms admitted to an inquisitive questioner that in the years since the oral contraceptive arrived in Britain, the average bra size had gone up from thirty-four to thirty-six. One large firm was astounded to discover that the demand for their large cup size in 1967 was double what it had been the year before. Perhaps the final proof that the pill had arrived was the announcement that, in the United States at least, the tax authorities had ruled that the cost of oral contraceptives could be held as a tax-deductible expense if it could be shown that another pregnancy would be a serious threat to a woman's health.

In the years since 1957, when the pill first became available, its use has increased at a rate the manufacturers, no doubt rightly, claim as triumphant proof of its acceptability. 'The pill is rapidly overtaking all other contraceptive methods as the most popular way to space children, limit family size or postpone a first pregnancy,' was the satisfied claim of one of the major pill-producing firms in February 1969. Figures from the Population Council in New York showed then that more than eighteen million women throughout the world were using oral contraceptives. Not only that, but the rate of use was increasing by thirty to forty per cent a year. It was predicted that by 1980 nearly 100 million women would be using this means of contraception.

Preference for the pill is highest in the developed countries, with more than nine million American women and one and a quarter million British women opting for it in 1969. One of the richest markets for the pill manufacturers has been Australasia, where 900,000 women, as it has been called, contracept orally – a figure that represents thirty-four per cent of the women of childbearing age. In that continent, it would seem, the pill is coming to be regarded as one of women's natural entitlements. In November 1969 a news sheet circulated among British drug firms reported that a bride-to-be who had hurt her leg in a car crash had been awarded £230 damages by a Melbourne court, because the risk of thrombosis would probably prevent her from ever taking the pill.

In Australia, the Minister for Health has said, contraceptive pills were becoming an important cause of accidental poisoning in young children – but it is a state of affairs not peculiar to that country. The Director of the Poisons Reference Service at Guy's Hospital, Dr Roy Goulding, said recently, 'Oral contraceptives must be present on half the kitchen tables of Britain judging by the number of children who stuff them down their throats.' Luckily, in Britain at least, no child has been known to die as a result, but this has not prevented the occasional panic when a box of contraceptive pills has been lost: police cars have been known to tour the streets uttering loudspeaker warnings about dangers to children, much to the annoyance of the pill's supporters, who point out that the worst that could befall a child who swallowed a whole month's supply, *pace* the Australian Health Minister, is that he would be sick. Meantime, women using the pill who hear the policemen's warning have their confidence weakened yet again.

Not every woman who starts to take the pill will go on doing so. When the extent of use of the pill was investigated in America in 1965, it was found that while 3·8 million women were actually taking it, another 2·5 million had taken it at some time, and more than half of those thought they would do so again. Some who stop taking it are 'natural' dropouts: they either want to have a baby or have passed the age when they can have one. But about eight in ten of those who stop, judging from the results of the National Fertility Survey in the USA in 1965, do so because of side-effects. In that study, of over 4,800 women under forty-five, one-third of those who had been on the pill at any time between 1960 and 1965 were not on it at the time of the survey.

In Cleveland, Ohio, a psychiatrist and a psychologist decided after studying the matter for four years that you could predict which women in any given sample would *not* persevere with oral contraception. It had very little to do with side-effects, they concluded: it was all in the mind. The ones who did persevere 'are generally more socially competent, self-satisfied and independent than the women who shifted to another form of contraception'. This conclusion was circulated with some satisfaction by the G. D. Searle Company, who added that the dropouts 'often paid a steep price for their uncertainty': thirty-three per cent of them had later had an unwanted pregnancy.

But whatever the reasons why users defect, the increasing numbers of pill patients are more than enough to compensate for them. In family planning clinics, more and more newly-enrolling patients are prescribed the pill, usually at their own request. If a girl attends a clinic and asks to be fitted with a diaphragm, some doctors at least tend to be on their guard. 'We are very much pill-oriented,' said a doctor working in a clinic in the Midlands. 'Our first choice would be the pill. And if they want anything else we want to know the reason why.' 'The cap is the thing their mother used,' said an experienced woman doctor in Surrey. 'And I seldom feel this is the normal thing to ask for. In fact it's abnormal not to want the pill.' In 1967 77,595 new patients at FPA clinics did want it – 5,644 more than the year before. What is more, the new patients were predominantly under thirty, and the ones between twenty and twenty-four formed the biggest and fastest-growing group of clients. 'Yes,' said the doctor in Surrey, 'the pill is definitely the young woman's contraceptive.'

In the report that carried the facts about new patients demanding the pill, the Family Planning Association emphasized that there was no evidence that giving the pill, or any other contraceptive, to the unmarried (as their clinics will do as a rule) increased sexual promiscuity in any age group.

But no matter how many times such a caution is repeated, there will be loud voices raised to the contrary. The pill has become an emblem of teenage permissiveness, like pot, pop music, long hair and unisex. To pessimists it is also an agent in the destruction of human dignity, and of what the Pope, in his 1968 Christmas message to the world, described as man's 'damnation by sensuality'.

'Society,' said the *Lancet* wisely in an editorial in 1969, 'wishes to prevent unintended conceptions by the most efficient means, but it fears the emergence of a generation which does not cherish chastity. Until society decides for itself the moral behaviour which it regards as acceptable, there is no clear guidance for the individual.' Typical of the kind of protest which greets the provision of better contraceptive advice to the young was the outraged reaction of a group of women in Newcastle-upon-Tyne when the FPA opened a birth control clinic for teenagers. Organizations claiming to represent more than 10,000 women, and linked with Anglican, Presbyterian, Catholic and Jewish groups, were quick to protest; a local woman magistrate and former city alderman said, 'We are all disgusted at the idea of our children being given contraceptives. It is time this country had a decent moral code for our young people to live by.'

There is nothing new about complaints of this kind, except that they now have the pill to focus upon. Protests against sexual licence and the collapse of traditional morality have always been part of the small change of public debate. Today they are reinforced by older people's reaction against the greater financial, moral and sexual independence of youth and the frightening pace of social change. The worst fears of those who condemn the pill on such grounds are confirmed when they read, for instance, letters like one that appeared in a Sunday newspaper from a single girl of twenty who had found it no problem to obtain a prescription for the pill from a private doctor. 'I can now see the complete psychological change I underwent during the six months I took it,' she confessed. 'Although I went on it purely for the sake of my boy friend, it became increasingly easy to stray from the path due to the total lack of inhibition. Promiscuity becomes as easy as another cigarette. In this respect the pill to the addict is as morally dangerous as heroin is physically.'

On the face of it, it might seem likely that the pill's availability has led to more acts of intercourse outside marriage. But it would be unwise to assume this is so without better proof than is usually forthcoming. The pill, after all, is hardly the ideal contraceptive for the casual fornicator: it is more often a precaution taken by couples who, in the usual phrase, have formed a stable relationship outside marriage.

This is borne out by numerous investigations which also strongly suggest that promiscuity – or greater sexual freedom – is happening independently of the development of new methods of birth control. Not only that, but the pill, which theoretically could lighten the consequences of promiscuity by reducing illegitimate births, is in fact not getting to the right people. The pill may be the young woman's contraceptive – but which young women? Not, apparently, the ones who need it most.

Many of the investigations into the extent of teenage sexual behaviour have been made among university students. It is not surprising: they are a cohesive, articulate, and statistically rather convenient group. What they lack in not being representative of youth as a whole, they make up in the sheer volume of what has been written about their sexual habits. These have been the subject of ever more illuminating and, to some, disturbing disclosures. In America, according to an estimate given to the 1968 convention of the American Medical Association by the eminent sociologist Professor Harold T. Christensen of Purdue University Indiana, nearly one-fifth of college girls and about half the boys, though unmarried, had had intercourse. The medical officer of the University College of South Wales told an international congress on mental health at around the same time that every year at his own college between ten and fifteen per cent of the unmarried girl students became pregnant: sexual problems, he remarked, were high on the list of student worries. 'Young people today,' he said, 'are allowing themselves far more sexual freedom. It is almost taken for granted that male and female students go to bed.' He was one of those who considered contraceptive advice should be provided for them, including the pill, if only because it made a useful regulator of menstruation at examination times. At Leeds University, a medical officer has said, 'If I know that there is an established relationship, and intercourse is taking place, I will prescribe it [the pill] rather than risk an unwanted pregnancy.' Figures showed that in one academic year, out of 2,226 women students there had been three hundred applications for the pill: yet forty-nine unmarried girls had become pregnant.

Not every student campus is as liberally supplied. A senior staff physician at the University of California said at a Washington meeting in 1967 that parents and other adults he had canvassed were unanimously against the dispensing of contraceptives to students. 'The college or university has a good reputation and moral image to maintain,' was his argument: supplying contraceptives would cause 'complete destruction of the moral ideas of marriage' and it was probably illegal as well. But another speaker at the same meeting, Dr Maurice M. Osborne Jr of Stanford University student health service, took a more lenient view: 'Physicians in general and college physicians in particular have ducked their responsibility in facing this very important preventive medical task – that is, the prevention of tragic instances of unwanted pregnancy, with the results ranging from premature and unstable marriages to illegal septic abortions, with results including death.' He went on to say that in many cases, although an unmarried girl appeared to want contraceptive advice or a prescription for the pill, 'she may really at a deeper level want to be encouraged and supported in her abstaining'. Counselling girls like these, Dr Osborne added, was 'one excellent method of contraception'.

The not-so-obvious motives of both men and women students in difficulties like these came under scrutiny in England from Dr Peter Gifford of Sheffield's student health service in 1968. The number of girls known to be pregnant had gone up from 0·7 per cent of the total number of students to 2·6 per cent in only two years, he found. In three out of ten, Dr Gifford considered, there was what he described as 'a neurotic wish to be pregnant'. Some of the men students involved felt parenthood to be a proof that they were adults, and used their girl friend's pregnancy as a weapon against people who wanted to treat them like children. And for some of the girls, pregnancy was a way of punishing their parents, their boy friends – or themselves. Some were even described as having 'a compulsive desire to be pregnant for pregnancy's sake'.

For whatever motives, one unmarried girl student in ten (it has been estimated from student health reports) becomes pregnant during her three years at a British university. Of these pregnancies, about two-thirds terminate in normal births and the rest in abortion. In itself this is one of the strongest arguments for providing some kind of regular contraceptive advice, and there is no question about the pill's advantages when it comes to choosing the appropriate contraceptive means. The point is illustrated at the Cambridge Advisory Centre for Young People, a clinic which dispenses birth control advice mainly to women undergraduates and girl friends of men undergraduates. One of its founders was Dr Malcolm Potts, then Director of Medical Studies at Sidney Sussex College. In the first two years of its existence (it was started in 1967) in a small converted house in the middle of Cambridge, the Centre enrolled 890 patients, and 88 of them were prescribed the pill. The other two were fitted with diaphragms and both became pregnant, a curiously high failure rate for this form of contraception. Both pregnancies ended 'after much trauma', according to Dr Shirley Emerson, in abortion.

Dr Emerson, a young and smartly dressed family doctor who is in practice nearby with her husband, is one of five doctors who run the clinic. The clients, she says, are all under twenty-five and all 'highly pill-conscious'. One of the most striking things about them is that taking the pill brings so few side-effects: 'They're not troubled by headaches or anything,' says Dr Emerson, 'and certainly not by lack of libido. To them sex is still an experiment, and a joy, not just a marital chore.'

She describes the girls at the Centre as intelligent and articulate, with a lot of questions to ask. Were they ever worried about the side-effects reported in the newspapers? 'They can appreciate the distinction between news reports and facts,' says Dr Emerson. 'In the first week of taking the pill they might feel dizzy or nauseated, and their periods might be a bit short, but this doesn't bother them at all.'

Dr Emerson has also noticed a conspicuous difference between the girls who attend the Centre and the older married women at another family planning clinic where she works some distance away. There, the patients' attitudes are complicated by the disappointments of their marriage and fear of failure in sexual relationships. 'People tend to have this tremendous psychological thing about orgasm,' Dr Emerson said.

'There are all these discussions about it, and how the done thing is to prove oneself sexually. There's a terrible fear of being frigid, and a feeling that there's something the matter with you if you don't have a full sexual experience. So they get married and have intercourse, but they won't admit to anyone except to themselves and the clinic that they're not enjoying it. Some women expect something absolutely ecstatic to happen when they cease to be virgins, and when it doesn't they are glad to be reassured they're normal. They get disillusioned, and come and have a groan: and this is I think why many doctors think women become depressed on the pill. I do see people who are perfectly happy, of course, they come for their pills and off they go. But some of them come to express dissatisfaction and they express it through the pill, often in terms of side-effects.'

Dr Malcolm Potts has analysed case histories of the first five hundred clients seen at the Cambridge advisory centre. The girls who used the Centre, he maintains, were not promiscuous, and many came with the boy friend with whom they were having or intending to have intercourse. (One in twelve of the girl clients were virgins.) 'The overwhelming majority of young people coming to us,' he has written, 'have established a stable relationship with one partner and we have observed that couples coming to the clinic see themselves as in love and intend to marry.'

However widespread the family planning gospel may appear to be, a closer look indicates otherwise. It re-emphasizes the need for a contraceptive as convenient and above all as efficient as the pill. Dr William Kind's survey mentioned just now indicated that in Leicester at any rate young people were less inclined to favour having intercourse with 'just anybody' than they had been five years earlier. This certainly applied to the girls, none of whom thought sex before marriage was justified 'with any consenting partner'. Twenty-two per cent of the men thought it was: but in 1963 thirty-nine per cent of the men had thought so and ten per cent of the girls. If there were 'special circumstances' this made a difference, and both men and women were ready to entertain the idea of sex before marriage if the partners were engaged or in order to 'deepen the relationship'. But surprisingly, whether or not contraceptives were used did not qualify as a 'special circumstance'. And, striking an even more disappointing note for family planning experts, sixty-eight per cent of the girls in 1968 thought sex without contraception was a chance worth taking – a twenty-five per cent increase on the previous survey.

But it is not only young unmarried girls who have so far failed to get the message about contraception. Thousands of couples in Britain still do not use even the most unreliable methods, let alone the pill. Instead they trust to luck. Of course, family planning specialists are well used to disillusionment: the birth control movement has had an uphill struggle from the start. Despite the publicity for birth control in general, and the pill in particular, the Family Planning Association had to live with the fact, in 1969, that seven per cent fewer people had any idea what the FPA did, compared with ten years before. The lower the social class, the less chance of the person knowing. It was some consolation that nearly three-quarters of the people in this poll approved of contraceptives being used in marriage, a big improvement over the fifty-seven per cent in 1959.

But it is debatable whether vague 'approval' of using contraceptives in marriage is enough. Among those who might well have said they approved, when asked the question by a girl from the poll organization standing at the door, could be Mr and Mrs G., the principal characters in a typical case history related by one health visitor at an FPA meeting. Their story illustrates some of the difficulties in the way of the family planning organizers. Both the G.'s were in their early thirties and neither was very bright. Mr G. was usually out of work. They had eight children, two of them at schools for the educationally subnormal and the rest under five at home. Both husband and wife agreed they did not want any more children, though they had no idea what to do about it. Mr G. insisted he was in charge and did not want his wife to see a doctor; but after a great deal of persuasion Mrs G. was finally escorted by the health visitor to a local family planning clinic. Mrs G. was put on the pill, but the health visitor who had followed their fortunes thus far called every day to remind her to take it. Nevertheless at the end of the first three months, Mrs G. did not go back for a new supply. Finally she agreed to have an intra-uterine device fitted, provided Mr G. agreed, and the tireless health visitor then had to visit the G.'s for several months to try to get him to sign a consent form – meantime keeping the couple supplied with condoms. At last the form was signed, the loop fitted, and when last heard of the G's had lasted two years without a pregnancy.

Stories like this could be told in hundreds of birth control clinics. Not all have the same optimistic ending. Wives are persuaded to accept the pill – which their husbands promptly throw on the fire. Patients hand their last week's supply of pills to the next door neighbour because they think she needs them more, or to a younger sister off for a weekend with a boy friend. Prescribing the pill is not enough: many women have to be told repeatedly how to take it, and not only have to be reminded to keep taking it but have their regular supply delivered to the door. In post-natal wards in hospital, gynaecologists and midwives who happen to be alert to the social needs of their patients make strenuous efforts to persuade them to plan the next child and not leave it to chance. Two gynaecologists writing in *The Practitioner* in August 1968 gave it as their opinion that about half the pregnancies occurring in Britain were 'basically unplanned'. 'Whilst the population explosion in other parts of the world constantly arouses our anxiety,' they warned, 'this acute problem is one which should also not be underrated at home.'

Their warning was not based on sheer impression, but on a questionnaire given to 1,500 patients at the obstetric booking clinics of two hospitals serving different types of community. By far the commonest reason for pregnancy was not that the couple had deliberately wanted a baby, but simply that no contraceptive precautions had been taken. This was so in seven out of ten pregnancies. In a large proportion of cases – seventeen per cent and twenty-five per cent respectively in the two hospitals – the woman had become pregnant despite the use of a contraceptive, including the pill.

Such figures are by no means unique, nor are they confined to England alone. A recent survey in Los Angeles in which interviewers spoke to nearly 1,300 women with families showed that eighty-four per cent of the primary school graduates among them had not planned their pregnancies. Seventy-two per cent of the high school graduates made the same admission and forty-three per cent of those with a college education. Sir Dugald Baird, Emeritus Professor of Obstetrics at Aberdeen University and a pioneer of enlightened birth control policies, concluded from a recent investigation that only forty per cent of the first babies in Scotland were planned. Even in Aberdeen itself, where thanks to Sir Dugald's efforts an unusually liberal attitude has been taken towards contraceptive needs, and towards abortion, twenty-five per cent of mothers in one study were found to have had more children after ten years of parenthood than they had said they wanted five years earlier. More than a quarter of the children born in the area, Sir Dugald has said, are 'unplanned and mostly unwanted', a circumstance which has cumulative social effects.

It could be, as has been suggested more than once, that taking a chance on pregnancy adds to the pleasure of intercourse. If so the effectiveness of the pill could be secretly disliked by some couples, and the family planning organizations have an even harder struggle than they thought. Luckily the days have gone when the workers in birth control clinics could be thought of as ineffectual enthusiasts leading a slightly ridiculous crusade for sexual freedom. Certainly not in Britain, where the clientèle at FPA clinics is on the increase. Some thousand clinics are now providing contraceptive advice, pills and appliances for nearly three-quarters of a million women of all social classes. New clinics are being opened at the rate of two or three a week while others, already in existence, are taken over by local authorities.

Under the Family Planning Act of 1967 birth control was placed on an official footing. Local authorities now have the power to make arrangements for family planning advice and appliances to be supplied to anyone who needs them, and they can give contraceptives free of charge at their discretion. In fact eighteen months after the Act (as the FPA noted at the time) only thirty-four out of 204 local authorities were providing a family planning service for everyone who wanted it, married or single; 129 were giving a restricted service, for instance providing the advice but not the supplies, or not advising the unmarried; thirty-nine authorities had either done nothing about the Act or were still talking about what they were going to do. Putting birth control on the map was evidently taking more than an Act of Parliament, and the FPA's Director, Mr Caspar Brook, dedicated the Association to a 'massive and sustained campaign' to persuade local authorities to put more money into family planning services.

In the vigorous growth of the FPA the pill has been an important factor. There was a time when birth control clinics were thought of as places where middle-class women could be fitted with diaphragms: working men used coitus interruptus or the condom – the cloth-cap contraceptive. But the middle-class image of the family planning clinic (no longer called the birth control clinic, or not officially) is disappearing, and it is largely because there is a practical, efficient, and 'aesthetically attractive' means of contraception: the pill. 'Women of all ages, with all family sizes from all social classes, are increasingly using the Family Planning Clinic,' stated a report from Aberdeen, which made it clear that the growing popularity of the establishment was due to oral contraceptives. Within a year of the pill's introduction there in 1964, three out of four newcomers to the clinic opted for oral contraception. By 1968 it was being prescribed for nine out of ten first attenders, with the occasional intra-uterine device or diaphragm being fitted for women apprehensive about 'taking hormones', or for those who had used the diaphragm before and were used to it. Moreover, most of the women already on the clinic's books had switched to the pill. The numbers attending the clinic rocketed. In three years they shot up from 2,261 to 6,432 – and the legitimate birth-rate slumped, from 3,073 to 2,580.

Yet the number of illegitimate pregnancies in Aberdeen had gone up by some twenty-three per cent in the same period. And as with Aberdeen, so with the nation. The 71,260 illegitimate pregnancies in England and Wales in 1967 represented a peak, over 10,000 more than in 1963. Easier abortion has since reduced the totals.

Of illegitimate births, some eighteen per cent are born to girls under twenty, a fact which affords unhappy confirmation of the conclusion reached by Dr William Kind in Leicester: these, no doubt, are the girls, or many of them, who thought intercourse without contraception a chance worth taking. Many of the others figure, one can assume, among the 72,595 shotgun marriages listed in the Registrar-General's returns for 1969, a group officially categorized as 'pre-maritally conceived legitimate live births'.

In the USA the same trend is visible. Ryder and Westoff, directors of the US National Fertility Survey, reported in 1967 an accelerating decline in fertility (not the same as a fall in population figures, which are going up) between 1960 and 1965.

The decline was paralleled by an increase in the use of the pill but, for various reasons, the two sociologists expressed their hunch that 'what has been happening to fertility in the nineteen-sixties would have happened in direction if not in degree even if the oral contraceptives had not appeared on the scene'. However, the tempo of decline in the later years of the survey, they considered, could probably be attributed in part to 'the availability of this highly efficient and apparently highly acceptable method of fertility regulation'.

But at the same time there appears to be a rise in the number of illegitimate births. One American bride in six is pregnant on her wedding day, the American Medical Association's annual convention for 1968 was told by Professor Harold T. Christensen, a man who it has been said has 'made almost a life-time endeavour' of his studies of child spacing and family planning. In New York in the same year, City Health Commissioner Dr Edward O'Rourke said, reviewing the state of the city's health, 'We have had 1,400 more births out of wedlock for January through October 1968, as compared with this period last year ... We had 20,238 out-of-wedlock births for the first ten months, January through October 1967. Now for this period in 1968, it is up to 21,656. And most of these babies are born in our poverty areas.' At least one baby in six born in the city was illegitimate and many of these were born to girls under eighteen.

Advice and exhortation about contraception given to girls like these would help to lighten the cumulative social problems their pregnancies cause. The growing custom enjoyed by places like the Brook Clinics in Britain, which specialize in contraceptive advice to unmarried girls, is an encouraging sign, except that like the Cambridge Advisory Centre, they tend to cater for the 'steady' couple who often have intercourse and presumably have gone to the clinic in a deliberate, premeditated attempt to make it safe to go to bed together.

Unfortunately the kind of sexual adventure which ends in illegitimate pregnancy is very often not at all premeditated. How could the pill help, when premeditation is exactly what it requires?

It has been suggested that the way out of the problem is to supply the pill as routine to all girls when they reach puberty. It is already being done in Baltimore, where girls in the ghetto areas without previous sexual experience are, according to a recent report, being given the pill. Some such just-in-case policy was evidently in the mind of a delegate who spoke at the 1967 Labour Party women's conference: urging that local authorities should extend their facilities for contraceptive advice, she declared, according to the report in *The Times*, 'The pill and the cervical coil were women's protection against one of the "increasing tragedies of the modern age" – enforced pregnancy by rape and sexual assault'.

Safety considerations seemed not to weigh too heavily on this speaker. Nor did they in the case of a Harvard nutritionist, Dr M. C. Latham, who wrote to the *British Medical Journal* in 1966 with the suggestion that in the future we might have 'a society where soon after the first onset of menstruation all females are fitted with an IUD'. The IUD and not the pill, he reasoned, because with oral contraceptives, and every other method of contraception, either husband or wife had to do something positive to prevent conception. Once in place, the intra-uterine device allowed unplanned and unlimited intercourse with no further contraceptive action, for years if need be. If a woman decided later on to have a baby, she would go to a clinic and have the device taken out: she would have to take a planned and deliberate step when she *did* want a baby, rather than when she did not.

Was it too extravagant an idea, Dr Latham wondered? 'I believe the benefits would far outweigh the disadvantages,' he said. 'Certainly if I had a daughter of sixteen I would happily have her fitted with such a device.'

Dr Latham's suggestion came a decade or two early. It was too much, at any rate, for several readers of the *Journal*, but their objections to it were not on the grounds of safety. What experience did Latham have of sexual neurosis, a retired psychiatrist from Pinner, Middlesex, wanted to know. 'From more than forty years' experience of these problems,' he stated, 'I cannot imagine any approach more likely to sow the seeds of the most intractable neuroses than Dr Latham's crude mechanistic approach to sex.' A Penzance anaesthetist, also retired, was reminded of the Weimar Republic and the proposal to march the high school girls down to be fitted with Graafenburg rings: an ominous precedent.

In their attitudes towards the social problems of abortion, sex before marriage, promiscuity and contraception doctors are as subject to prejudice as anyone else. An understanding of the anatomy and physiology of sex does not automatically confer any depth of understanding of its emotional burdens, as many a patient has had to learn in an embarrassed colloquy with his or her doctor. The pill has done a lot to make discussion of contraception socially acceptable, but the fact seems to have taken some doctors by surprise. And as a conservatively inclined profession, doctors are in some danger of being left behind in a period of rapid liberalization of sexual behaviour. As it is, their public reputation is of a somewhat reactionary body, not keen, for example, on abortion law reform and more worried about upholding conventional morality than attending to the medical consequences of flouting it.

At a meeting of the International Planned Parenthood Federation in Copenhagen in 1966, Sir Theodore Fox, formerly Editor of the *Lancet*, addressed himself to the subject of 'educating the educators', a category in which the average doctor, whether he welcomes it or not, increasingly finds himself when it comes to the patient's sexual problems. The contraceptive revolution, he said, had made it possible not only to accept teenage sexual experimentation but to protect young people from its unwanted result, namely pregnancy. Premarital intercourse could be damaging to young people or it could be beneficial. 'Personally I believe that we must leave them to decide whether to try the experiment,' said Sir Theodore, 'but on two conditions only. They must have enough knowledge to know – and if possible understand – what they are doing to each other and to themselves. And they must always use effective contraceptives, which at present they very plainly do not.' A little later Dr Alex Comfort, commenting that others beside juveniles were in need of sexual education, recounted an incident when some boys were accused before Nottingham Juvenile Court of having intercourse with girls under age, allegedly at the girls' suggestion. One boy was sent to an attendance centre after hearing the magistrate declare, 'This was deliberate misbehaviour on your part because you carried and used contraceptives.'

But in general Sir Theodore's level-headed argument evoked criticism of a familiar type. A psychiatrist from Worcester wrote: 'At present our women are paying an enormous price for sexual freedom in unwanted pregnancies, abortions, forced marriages, venereal disease and personal humiliation.' No doubt, he remarked ironically, Sir Theodore felt these dangers could be avoided by education.

Some of them, though the doctor did not say so, could have been avoided by contraception. The exception is venereal disease. The swift rise in the number of cases of VD in the last few years has given armchair moralists a handy new weapon with which to chastise the young. It has also fanned into life what in the fifties was a dying medical speciality. 'Anyone who contemplates a career in venereology these days,' I remember a doctor telling the Council of the BMA in 1958, 'must be a super-optimist.' Now, for venereologists the world over, the subject is undergoing what one London specialist called a spectacular renaissance. Dr Robert Catterall, at the Middlesex Hospital's venereology department in London, noted recently that a hundred million new gonorrhoea infections occurred throughout the world every year. In America, venereologists are using phrases like 'spiralling to epidemic levels' and 'spreading like a prairie fire' to describe the increase in venereal disease. The American Social Health Association's National Survey of VD Incidence (a government-backed inquiry) shows an annual rate of increase, for gonorrhoea, of between 12 and 15 per cent over the past five years. The latest figure – for 1969 – of 494,000 new cases reported is believed by the ASHA to be only about one quarter of the actual total.

As for infectious syphilis, this had been on the decline until 1970 – when the figures suddenly showed an 8½ per cent increase, an increase 'so dramatic that national emergency action is needed', the ASHA said. And again, the reported figures are believed to underestimate the true incidence.

In Britain, no similar resurgence in the syphilis figures has yet been reported. But the incidence of gonorrhoea during the 1960s rose by nearly 24 per cent. A number of reasons have been put forward to account for this. For one thing venereal diseases have long been notorious for their ability to make a comeback after apparently fading away. Again although the organism that causes syphilis is still sensitive to antibiotic drugs, the gonococcus increasingly is not. Another possible factor is immigration and the presence in large cities of numerous home-sick men, as well as the greater frequency with which people travel. Interviewed by a medical magazine in 1969 Dr Catterall instanced the case of a businessman who flew to Sydney where on his first night he got drunk and slept with a hostess. From there he flew on to San Francisco and did the same thing. Next he went to New York, picked up a girl, but decided against sleeping with her because he found it was painful to pass water. By the time he arrived back in London and turned up at the Middlesex Hospital, he was an established case of gonorrhoea. The assumption was that he had picked up the disease from the girl in Sydney and passed it on to the girl in San Francisco, who by the time he reached home had probably infected several other men.

Whatever the situation in the business community, once again the student population has come in for special scrutiny. In Sheffield, from 1961 to 1965, the members of the student body who attended 'special clinics' (VD clinics) went up from 2·9 per thousand to 5·5. Nearly half the men and twenty-eight per cent of the girls who attended had venereal or some other sexually transmitted disease. A local venereologist attributed it to, among other things, the fact that many more students than in the past were the first generation in their families to go to a University and, as he put it, 'have perhaps been less exposed to traditional middle-class ways of thinking about sex'. It was not clear from this comment who had been influenced by whom.

In all the speculation about the most likely explanation for the increase in VD, the pill not surprisingly figures prominently – usually because it is assumed to encourage promiscuity. In fact the number of known cases of gonorrhoea was increasing in Britain before the pill became available in 1961. Promiscuity was also being given as one of the main causes then. But there is another way in which the pill might be implicated: it provides no protection against transmission of the gonorrhoea microbe. Condoms or, as the manufacturers prefer to call them, protectives to some extent do. 'The pill will not kill the gonococcus or the dreaded *T.pallidum* of syphilis,' wrote a retired immunologist from Sussex to the *British Medical Journal* in 1968. With scarcely-concealed distaste, he went on: 'The more primitive, but safer, sheath at least afforded some protection against these and other infections. People with free ideas on sexual intercourse, whether they rely on the pill or not as a contraceptive, are very likely to contract venereal disease and communicate it to their existing paramour.'

But besides the lack of any barrier against the gonococcus, there is also some suspicion that women who use oral contraceptives are more susceptible to venereal infection. The evidence is not conclusive, but it has been suggested that the cells of the cervical canal become more receptive to infection in a woman who is taking the pill. It is also possible that a woman's immunity to infection might be weakened by the altered hormonal environment.

Should the point be proved, one cannot help foreseeing a certain grim satisfaction on the part of some of the pill's antagonists whose objections to it are moral rather than scientific. Contraception, after all, like the venereal infections as a group, belongs in that contentious region where morality and medical practice get mixed up. In his book *The Anxiety Makers*, published in 1967, Dr Alex Comfort illustrates convincingly the way doctors have manufactured public anxiety in support of accepted morality, threatening dire consequences to health as a result of masturbation and sexual intercourse – especially adulterous intercourse. The high point of that 'flood of motivated nonsense about every aspect of sexual hygiene which flowed over the public from authoritative scientific sources', Comfort observes, was the nineteenth century. But some of the admonitions uttered then were echoed in some of the public pronouncements, freighted with gloom, made by doctors in the sixties.

The voice of the anxiety-maker made itself heard very soon after the pill's arrival on the medical scene. Hardly had the first Englishwoman begun to take it than a Manchester surgeon was writing to the *Lancet*:

Although long threatened I hope some others groaned to learn from the daily press that an oral contraceptive had reached clinical trial in Birmingham ... This method of birth control contains two offences against humanity which other methods do not have. The first offence is suppression of normal physiological function. The method secondly offends by not being an open and unconcealed contract between the parties. It is possible that either the man or woman could see that the pill is given surreptitiously without consent or knowledge of the other, or worse, it could be given by an outside agent either for public or private purposes. These are basal offences which it is difficult to reconcile with any code of morals hitherto held in this end of Europe ... It seems to me that a profession which is prepared to handle this drug in this country is betraying a sacred heritage. The opportunity is still open – refuse to handle it, before it is too late.

It was already too late, of course. The idea of a grand medical boycott of the pill to prevent, say, its underhand use dissolved in the morning tea, was and is a doomed hope. Yet from time to time grave headshaking goes on in medical circles, seeming to reflect a greater concern over the moral implications of oral contraception than one would expect. Discussing the problem of student promiscuity the *British Medical Journal* adopted a magisterial I-mention-no-names tone probably intended to make one or two student health doctors feel uncomfortable:

In spite of denials in some quarters, most people who stop to think would agree that sexual promiscuity is debasing to the personalities of those who practise it, fraught with serious dangers, especially to women, and damaging to the interests of society.

The statistics of pregnancy and venereal disease among students made the writer wonder

whether universities and colleges are doing all they should to educate, in the fullest sense the students in their charge. The remedy
advocated by some people – namely, the provision of contraceptives
to the young on request – is not without its own hazards ... To
prescribe oral contraceptives may reduce the risk of an unwanted
pregnancy and relieve anxiety on this score, but it may also increase
the inner conflicts that can arise from a guilty conscience and do a
real disservice to the student.

It is hard to tell how much of this sententiousness spills over
into the normal traffic of information between the patient and
the doctor in his surgery. Not much perhaps. But the evidence
is that, for whatever reason, a far from negligible proportion of
family doctors in Britain try to avoid the subject of contraception when talking to their patients. When Dr Ann Cartwright,
of the Institute of Community Studies, ran her survey of nearly
two thousand doctors and their attitudes to family planning
advice in 1968 she discovered that not even special circumstances would make some of them discuss the subject with their
patients. Just over ten per cent of them would not, for instance,
discuss it with an unmarried woman who had just had a baby,
even if the woman asked for advice, presumably taking this
attitude on moral grounds. But one in two thousand of the doctors said they would not talk about family planning even if they
were asked directly by a married woman with two children and
a heart condition which would make another pregnancy extremely dangerous. And one in two hundred would have
changed the subject if a married woman with three children,
and only one bedroom, asked them for advice. Taking these
latter two results into account, Dr Cartwright remarked: 'Even
if the percentages are low it still means that for a number of
married women in England and Wales – probably more than
65,000 under forty-five – their GPs are just not prepared to discuss family planning.' Most of the doctors would help, of
course, though it took a variety of hypothetical situations for
them to do it. As to what action the doctors took: prescribing
the pill, Dr Cartwright noted, was much the commonest action
taken – only one in twenty of the doctors never did so.

It also emerged from this investigation that family doctors

are playing an increasing part in advising patients about family planning: a similar survey five years earlier had shown that only half the GPs questioned thought it was their job to give contraceptive advice; now, sixty-seven per cent thought so. The snag is that the majority of doctors have never had any training in giving advice about sexual problems, contraception included. Few medical schools include family planning and guidance on sexual problems in their courses. The cost of the omission is borne by many an anxious patient. 'Many of us are painfully aware,' Dr Jean Pasmore said at a meeting in September 1968 to discuss relations between patients and GPs, 'that our basic medical training does not give us much help in treating our patients' emotional and sexual problems.' Dr Pasmore, who runs a 'marital clinic' at a hospital on the outskirts of London, illustrated her point with a patient's description of how a doctor dealt with her sexual problems: 'We went to our doctor when we got back from our honeymoon because we couldn't manage it, and he said to take me out and give me one or two drinks and we'd be all right. We did try that but it was no good, so we didn't go back. That was two, four, eight years ago, and now I'm over thirty and do so want a family . . .' Another patient had said: 'I told my doctor I didn't get anything out of it, but he said lots of women are like me, so I've just put up with it all these years . . .'

In the USA a similar want of understanding seems to prevail. In 1968 a sociologist, Dr David R. Mace, told the American Medical Association (AMA) that all reliable evidence showed that American doctors were 'floundering rather helplessly' when faced with patients who had sexual problems. And in the following year, the AMA's Clinical Convention in Denver, Colorado, was given a lecture by Professor Kermit E. Krantz of the University of Kansas Medical Centre. 'We as physicians are leaders of the team,' Professor Krantz declared, 'and we're hung up on sex. We've been hung up a long time. We've divided people into two portions : above and below the navel. We want nothing to do with what goes on below the navel. What we know is that we've been taught that sex and marriage are synonymous.' The meeting also heard Dr Alan F. Guttmacher say that approximately one in three American women of fertile age were now using the pill and that whether his audience liked it or not, a sexual revolution was under way among the young. 'We are not going to change it,' said Dr Guttmacher. 'What is more, the new generation is a damned good one. In their sexual patterns they are not promiscuous. We can't turn the clock back. What shall we, therefore, do? Punish the kids by letting the girls get pregnant?'

It could be argued that the very existence of the Family Planning Association is a sign of the failure of the majority of family doctors, over the years, to give advice on an important branch of social medicine and the personal problems of the patient. Likewise the short existence of the organization known as Step One is, or was, another reproach to the GP in Britain. Step One, operating from an address in South London, maintained a list of doctors 'willing to discuss contraceptive problems in a friendly and helpful manner, and ready to prescribe the pill, or where the pill is not suitable, to provide other contraceptive advice'. Their roster of sympathetic GPs contained nearly two hundred names, in fifty-seven towns: anyone who answered their advertisement and sent £2.00. would be supplied with the name and address of a doctor living conveniently near. 'Don't be shy about approaching the doctor we have chosen for you,' was Step One's advice to its clients. 'It is quite ethical for him to prescribe the pill.' Unfortunately, if the girls were not shy, many of the doctors were, and wrote indignantly to Step One demanding that their names be removed from the list. The names had been chosen by a method described as a trade secret but the selection could not have been very careful: some of the doctors proved not at all sympathetic to the single girls who were encouraged to use this unique service, and some were Roman Catholics. Step One went out of business.

The fact that some of the doctors whose names were circulated by Step One were Roman Catholics would not necessarily mean they would refuse to prescribe the pill or give some other form of contraceptive advice. For all its explosive impact when published in the summer of 1968 the Papal encyclical *De*

*Humanae Vitae*, reaffirming Vatican opposition to birth control, has evidently made little difference to the prescribing habits of Roman Catholic doctors or to contraception among Catholic patients. A public opinion poll published after the encyclical showed that only a minority of Catholics in Britain supported the Pope's ruling. The great majority of those who had been using the pill or other methods of birth control intended to go on doing so. Also there was a strong suspicion among the interviewers who worked on the survey that, because of their reluctance to criticize the Pope, some Catholics were a good deal less happy about the encyclical than they claimed. 'It is possible,' said the report, 'that the figures may actually overstate the size of the minority.'

A similar story was told in the findings of the Population Investigation Committee, in 1969, based on interviews with over 2,300 British women who were questioned about their attitudes to and experience of birth control. Nearly eighty per cent of the Catholic women had used various methods at some time in their marriages (the actual figure, 78·3 per cent, compares with 87·4 per cent among all women). Coitus interruptus was even more favoured among the Catholics than the non-Catholics. And 16·4 per cent of all women had used the pill. Understandably, very many more Catholics than non-Catholics used the rhythm method, restricting intercourse to those times in the month when it is supposed to be safe, and according to Catholic dogma the only method which is in accordance with natural design. In fact, besides being notoriously unreliable, the rhythm method is believed by some to be responsible for a slightly higher incidence of deformed births among Catholic mothers, because more conceptions take place later in the cycle, with ova which have passed their prime.

In the USA the same picture emerges of surreptitious flouting of official Church teaching. And a massive review of the influence of Catholic principles on contraceptive practice all over the world, compiled in 1968 by two staff members of the Population Council, New York, showed that the general pattern was repeated throughout the developed countries. There were plenty of gaps in the survey. The authors could discover almost nothing about the large Catholic populations of Italy and Spain and had very little information on rural Latin America. Nor was there enough information about Catholics 'according to degree of religiosity': but it was evident that, for instance, Catholics in developed regions were closer to their non-Catholic countrymen in their attitudes to birth control than they were to members of the same Church in the undeveloped countries. In short, Catholics in the developed countries practise contraception widely, and although they rely to a greater extent on the rhythm method, most of them have used methods which are inconsistent with the principles of their religion. Those methods include the pill, and they also include abortion, a method even more repugnant to their Church. And not only do the majority of Catholics think the Church's opinion on birth control ought to be revised, but the number who hold this view, including the more devout, is increasing all the time.

As one could expect, general approval of large families by the Roman Catholic church (or, as the Population Council put it, the 'pro-fertility impact of Catholicism') makes for larger sized average families among Catholics than non-Catholics, and the family size ostensibly regarded as ideal by Catholics is higher. But in the undeveloped countries, the high rate of fertility among all families, regardless of religion, blots out any differences between Catholics and non-Catholics. Even so, city life in such countries means more contraception. In the large cities of Latin America the proportion of Catholics who use birth control methods, including forbidden ones, is higher than in any other of the poorer countries. Torn between the instructions of the priest and the doctor, a woman who has already experienced the freedoms of the pill usually prefers to be guilty of a technical transgression. Dr Edris Rice-Wray, at Mexico City's Maternal Health Association, went to the trouble of printing comments from more than fifty Catholic mothers a few weeks after the Papal encyclical. These are some of them:

'Well, like my husband says, "Pray to God and go to Mass, but keep taking the pills because if we have any more children the Pope isn't going to give us a hand to educate them."'

'I would like to use rhythm but don't understand it. My

neighbour uses it and she already has two daughters. I confessed and the Father would not forgive me for using the pills. I told him that for me it was much more of a sin to have an abortion or have my children before time so that they die soon after birth. The priests say no to birth control because they don't care when the children die. I think what I am doing is right.'

'Look Miss, I am a Catholic but even though the Pope will never forgive me I won't pay attention to what he said. Even when my friends say, "Graciela, stop taking the pills, don't you know what the Pope said." I tell them that I am Catholic and even if the Pope excommunicates me I will keep taking the pills because if I don't keep satisfying my husband he'll go off with another woman and leave me and my children without a crumb . . .'

Four years after publication the sum effect of the 1968 encyclical appears to have been not a fall in pill sales but a nearly irreconcilable division in the Roman Catholic church. On the side of those Roman Catholics who stand by the pill is Dr John Rock, one of the original quadrumvirate who pioneered the pill's clinical use. Now turned eighty, he is still working in Boston ('I've lost count of how many coronaries I've had,' he said) as Director of the Rock Reproductive Clinic, an institution described in its literature as 'for diagnosis and treatment, clinical and basic research, teaching, relating to sex and particularly to control of conception, with equal attention to infertility and inappropriate fertility'. The language of the Clinic's brochure, as can be seen, tends towards the statesmanlike, with the matter of contraception placed firmly in perspective with other, less controversial activities. Rock was long ago able to satisfy himself that his work on contraception was justified, arguing that the pill was an adjunct to nature, although it was easier for Catholics to settle their consciences before *De Humanae Vitae* appeared, reiterating a judgement on the subject which many Catholics hoped the pill would modify. After the encyclical Rock confessed he was 'surprised and unhappy' but was unwilling to change his own attitude. He believed the Pope was 'failing in his job' in writing the disputed document, which in his opinion states 'a position no longer valid and purely traditional, at a time when the Church has publicly absolved Galileo of his misjudged so-called error in declaring that the earth revolves round the sun. 'We can't wait another 300 years,' he said, 'for the Church to admit it's made another mistake when we're dealing with something like population.' He also believes Catholics who want to practise birth control will not be much affected by the encyclical: but 'it just might increase their guilt a little'. In some of his public comments Rock has gone further than this, telling one inquirer that he was not only surprised, but 'scandalized': 'Given the transparency of the requirements of mankind, one hardly expected the avowed leader of Christianity to abdicate so completely responsibility for the ultimate welfare of all.' But he said he was not embittered, still regarded himself as a Catholic and did not think he was going to be 'kicked out'. 'I have utter and complete confidence in the Catholic Church,' he said. 'I believe it could be about as dependable a transmitter of the mind of God as man can evolve. And until I see better, I stand by this one.'

On 22 August 1968, less than a month after publication of the encyclical, Pope Paul arrived for a three-day visit to Colombia, in the course of which he urged the Latin-American bishops to do all in their power to ensure that his ban on contraceptives was carried out. But hardly had the Pope returned to Rome before the Presidents of the Academies of Medicine from seven Latin-American countries, most of them with a predominantly Catholic population, met, also in Bogota, Colombia. The joint declaration issued at the end of their three-day meeting stressed the importance of maintaining and extending planned parenthood campaigns which made use of 'scientific methods selected with adequate medical and social considerations'. The seven doctors declared that the demographic problem in their countries was caused especially by the accelerating growth of population, and the limits this placed on the development of natural resources.

The world's population problem is grave enough to take much of the force out of not only *De Humanae Vitae*, but many of the objections to the pill on grounds of safety. Fifteen years ago the problem was no more than a cloud on the horizon to all but a few clairvoyant scientists. Since then the threat has grown more and more horrendous – and inescapable, with demographers and biologists making ever more spine-chilling forecasts of what is going to happen unless the relentless increase is halted. Standing-room only on the earth, suggested a *New Scientist* contributor not long ago, with the oceans floored over and all natural beauty obliterated, and the wretched inhabitants of honeycomb dwellings fed through tubes with their own (processed) excreta and forbidden to move more than a few feet in case they generate too much warmth. Other population experts say it is unlikely that we shall ever reach this stage: before that happened, we should have been roasted in a thermo-nuclear exchange, or stricken by world-wide infectious plague caused by not only over-population but 'ecocatastrophe' – irreversible degeneration in the quality of our environment. Public response to this seems slow. Apathy is probably the natural reaction to a situation that passed long ago out of the individual's control. But the population problem will not go away if we do not look, and next to the kind of statistics that demographers display before numbed newspaper readers, the efforts of planned parenthood organizations seem puny indeed. At a symposium organized in autumn 1969 by the Institute of Biology in Britain, Professor Paul R. Ehrlich of Stanford University warned his audience, 'Governments, including eventually a world body, must undertake the task of regulating the population size, just as they now attempt to regulate economies.' One possibility, he suggested, was the use of mass fertility-reducing agents, administered to whole populations. Meantime, research into what could be done by way of compulsory birth control ought to go ahead at top speed.

In Britain it is likely to take some time for a policy of this sort to be accepted. At the same symposium a Ministry of Technology official argued that there was no case for an active population policy in Britain in view of the uncertainties of prediction and the country's comparatively insignificant population explosion. An extra twelve million by the year 2000, which is the projection currently made for the likely increase in this country, does not seem much compared with the extra people, the equivalent of whole new continents, expected to be born elsewhere. This comfortable thought soon withers with the realization that with more people to feed in the countries from which we get our food, Britain will be increasingly thrown back on her own inadequate natural resources. The annual birth-rate in Britain is falling, temporarily at least. It reached a peak in 1964 and then began to fall away; but it is expected to rise again during the next few years because the number of women in the main child-bearing age group – the twenties – is rising sharply as a consequence of the higher birth-rate of the forties. One encouraging trend, incidentally, detected by a leading geneticist, Dr Cedric Carter, is that people in high-intelligence occupations, typically self-employed professional men, are now having, on average, larger families than almost any other group in the community. The trend can be discovered from analysing official census figures, says Dr Carter, who is Director of the Medical Research Council's Clinical Genetics Research Unit, but he has confirmed it by a private survey among former scholars of Winchester, who averaged more than three children apiece: among those who had become Fellows of the Royal Society the average went up to four a head, and the top of the table was occupied by a Nobel Prizewinner who was father of eight.

The birth-rate has fallen slightly in America, too, and it is tempting to attribute the general decline in fertility in the affluent West (not the same as a decline in overall population figures) to the fact that better contraceptives are available. This may well be the reason. But the obvious explanation is not necessarily the true one. Changes in the birth-rate have happened in various countries and at various times in history independently of the existence of efficient birth control methods. As Peter Fryer points out in his book *The Birth Controllers*, at the end of the eighteenth century and the beginning of the nineteenth the birth rate in France (where the main contraceptive device was the vaginal sponge, soaked in various solutions – sometimes brandy and water) fell from 38·6 per thousand to 31·3 – and by the eighteen-seventies it was 25·4. Fryer attributes this decline to Frenchwomen's wish to avoid unhealthily frequent pregnancies, to economic anxiety, and a greater respect for children. More recently, in the nineteen-thirties, the birth-rate in America fell – at a time of economic instability and before anyone had thought of the now voguish phrase 'contraceptive technology'. If the motivations are strong enough, it seems the effect desired by demographers can be produced; and if it can be done with nothing more sophisticated than the devices used by the great seducers of history (Casanova favoured the condom), one may wonder whether the pill really is, as is frequently claimed, the only way of defusing the population explosion.

As a means of controlling population in poor and deprived countries the pill has disadvantages. Although its cost is frequently subsidized, it is expensive, compared with, for instance, intra-uterine devices, which cost a few pennies each. And its use requires a certain amount of understanding of what the pill is doing, so that the woman can follow the three-weeks-on, one-week-off regimen. In this respect, the 'mini-pill', with its convenient everyday dosage, was an improvement. In fact when the Population Council in New York surveyed the use of oral contraceptives in the developing countries at the end of 1967, they reported that, while the use of the pill throughout the world had almost doubled in the two and a half years to July 1967, in the developing countries it had almost quadrupled. But continuation rates tend to be higher in the developed than the undeveloped countries: women in India and Malaya leave off taking the pill (and may or may not change to another method of birth control) sooner than women in Britain or America, and a substantial portion of the dropouts, especially in the first three months of use, discontinue because of side-effects. The report implied that the better educated and better off the women are, the longer they stay with oral contraceptives. But in Korea and Taiwan, and possibly in other countries as well for which statistics are not available, introduction of the pill into family planning programmes made no difference to the numbers of women starting to use IUDs in the programmes' early months, so that the total number of people who accepted some form of birth control went up. As the price of the pill went down, the Population Council found, more women began to take it, more of them stayed on it, and the proportion accepting the IUD in competition with the pill decreased.

The fact that IUDs have been widely used in underdeveloped countries has tended to give these devices the reputation of being the contraceptive method for poor and relatively unintelligent women. This is not so at all, according to the man who probably knows more about the history, and present and future use of the IUD than anyone, Dr Christopher Tietze, of the Population Council's Bio-Medical Division. He points out that world-wide use of IUDs now stands at about half the rate of oral contraceptive use: somewhere around eight million, with perhaps three million of these women in the USA. These, however, are figures for the number of IUDs supplied. 'We have no idea how many are in place in the United States,' Tietze told me, 'almost certainly more than one and less than two million. How many are on the shelf, in wholesalers', retailers', and doctors' offices, how many are in the uterus, and how many down the drain – I do not know.' As for American women regarding the IUD as the peasant's contraceptive, Tietze said: 'This is by no means true. A woman who pays seventy-five dollars for an insertion may be stupid – but she certainly isn't poor.'

IUDs at least have a longer history than oral contraceptives, because something rather like them was first used, in Britain, in the eighteen-sixties. They are devices (now made of plastic, or sometimes stainless steel) inserted into the womb and left there – and they may stay for years at a time. They come in various shapes – bow, ring, coil, loop, wishbone, clover leaf and comet-shaped (a ring with a tail). No finally agreed explanation has been put forward of how they work, but they do not prevent ovulation and the effect is presumably a local one. The reported side-effects include heavy and irregular bleeding, backache, cramps, and abdominal pain, though they are almost as efficient contraceptively as the pill, with a failure-rate of around 2.5 in every hundred woman-years. One of the major problems, however, is that IUDs are often involuntarily expelled from the womb (in some studies as many as thirty per cent came out) and the woman may not know this has happened: this is one reason why IUDs with tails were produced, so that there is an easy way to check that the device is still in position.

The cheapness and convenience of IUDs make them probably the strongest competitor to the pill so far in the world population stakes – IUDs, and, probably, male sterilization. Sterilization has the advantage of being one hundred per cent efficient, provided the couple take care to use some other contraceptive for the first few months, but has the disadvantage of being to all intents and purposes a final solution to the birth control problem. Not even the Simon Population Trust, which has done a great deal to popularize male sterilization by putting men who want the operation in touch with a surgeon who will do it, can say exactly how many men have had a vasectomy in Britain. The number runs into many thousands, but because the operations are usually done privately there is no official record of the numbers. In Britain it has been estimated that about twenty thousand women are sterilized every year: it is a great deal easier for women to have the operation under the National Health Service, but it is only a matter of time before it will be equally easy for men to have vasectomies without having to pay the surgeon. (In 1970 it became possible for men to have the operation under the NHS, 'in the interests of the health of either husband or wife', Mr Richard Crossman told the House of Commons.) In America, about 45,000 men are sterilized for contraceptive purposes every year, compared with some 65,000 women.

One of the reasons why the desire to have a vasectomy has not yet spread like wildfire among men in the West is that the operation is virtually irreversible. The suggestion has been made several times that deep-freezing techniques should be used to store a man's sperm before he has the operation done, so that if he should ever want to father another child, the means to do so could be, as it were, taken down from the laboratory shelf, thawed, and used by a process of artificial insemination. When Tietze and two other research workers from the National Committee on Maternal Health interviewed seventy-three men who had been sterilized, they found that all but one of them said they would do it again if they had the choice, and only two would not recommend it to others. But there was distinct evidence that quite a large proportion of the men had emotional reservations. Only thirty-five of the men actually had recommended the operation to someone else, and when they were asked if they cared if other people knew they had been sterilized, many of them 'flinched and showed tension', even if they answered 'no' to the question. 'It seemed clear that most men assumed a loss of status attendant upon sterilization,' said the paper in which these results were given. Although the men were willing to deal with their own doubts, they were not so ready to face the disapproval of others. The men's comments were: 'People think it's a form of castration and affects potency.' 'My brother-in-law thought it unmanly, my Catholic friends said, "How could you?"' 'My brother said, "If I had one, I'd turn into a fairy. In a few years, I wouldn't have any organs left."'

When a research worker from the London School of Hygiene and Tropical Medicine, Helen Wolfers, tried to measure the 'psychosocial and sexual effects' of vasectomy, she found that ten out of eighty-two Swindon men whom she questioned had some form of psychological problem arising from the operation. Some complained of being relatively impotent compared with before the vasectomy, some were depressed, some had found their existing troubles with premature ejaculation had become worse. Miss Wolfers believed that anyone who already had marriage problems should be dissuaded from having the operation and (in a *British Medical Journal* paper) made the familiar call for further investigation into the matter. Such is the growing interest in the operation as a means of contraception, the sooner more research is done the better.

Tietze remarks that the instinctive feeling that sterilization and castration are the same thing is strongly held among American and British men, but that in India this does not appear to be so. By 1970 the total number of sterilizations carried out in India was, officially, over five and a half million, about fifty per cent of the total world figure. Something like ninety per cent of the operations were performed on men, and the Population Council has spoken of the increasing popularity of the method all over India, even including rural areas. The result has been achieved by all kinds of stratagems including what is known (and it might have been better if they had chosen another name for it) as the 'camp approach'. In fact this means setting up sterilization camps at central points to serve a collection of nearby villages (in one camp in the state of Andhra Pradesh more than 2,300 women had the operation known as tubectomy before the camp packed up and moved off to another strategic site).

This idea is only one part of the 'cafeteria' system developed in India in an attempt to win over to contraception nearly a hundred million eligible couples. These couples can, if they want to, pick and choose between every available method of contraception which has a reasonable chance of curbing unwanted births. Even the rhythm method is on offer, along with condoms, foam tablets, jellies, diaphragms and IUDs – and, of course, though to a limited extent, the pill. Astonishing ingenuity has been used to try to popularize birth control. The ideas introduced with the encouragement of the ebullient Minister of Health Dr Sirpati Chandrasekhar include using elephants decorated with birth control slogans, who hand out condoms to passers-by with their trunks. And if on the Indian continent a man gets talking to another passenger on a train and brings the conversation round to sex, the chances are he could be a government-employed 'motivator', one of a number (some of whom make railway trains their hunting ground) hired to spread the family planning gospel, not necessarily because they believe in it but, as Tietze remarked, because they see the opportunity to make a fast rupee. Motivators, or canvassers, in India get ten rupees for every case they bring forward to a surgical clinic that is accepted for a vasectomy: this incentive payment has led to the organization of 'firms' by individual canvassers, who use agents to locate cases and see them through the operation. Some city hospitals have more than a hundred agents working with the canvasser, and the agents get half the fee. The system has had its abuses: sometimes the canvassers have forged the wife's signature on the vasectomy consent form, some have brought along technically ineligible bachelors to be sterilized and some have swindled the patients out of all or part of the compensatory grant of thirty rupees paid to them. Some canvassers have been reported to be making exorbitant incomes by inflating their returns of the number of operations performed.

All this has cast doubt on the official figures rendered to the international agencies, and demographers are beginning to suspect that India's progress in controlling the birth rate is slower than it would seem. However, Dr Chandrasekhar, a self-confessed optimist, has said that by 1974 they should have succeeded in reducing the birth rate by about one-fifth. (At present the Indian population increases every year by about the size of the population of Australia.) As he travelled round the country, he said in a BBC broadcast in 1969, he was struck with the impression that family planning propaganda had reached saturation point. Everywhere – on buses, billboards, on every vacant wall-space in towns and villages – could be seen the emblem of the Indian family planning movement, the red triangle.

In Pakistan equally novel ideas have been tried. In one area in East Pakistan publicity and information were brought to the people by a singing team who were recruited from local performers and who composed songs in the local idiom, often in a question-and-answer form which stressed the economic and family health advantages of contraception.

Although these energetic efforts are beginning to have some effect on the birth-rate in these countries, the pill itself has not had as much to do with it as other methods of contraception. Pakistan is one of those countries which have yet to take to the pill: there, the IUD is the method used in official family planning programmes. In India, the pill is being tried in a series of experimental, demonstration projects, but the total number of Indian women who use oral contraceptives is probably less than a quarter of a million. Its effectiveness is not in doubt: but it is hard to make sure the women take it regularly and that they have regular medical examinations.

Elsewhere in the world the pill has, to a greater or lesser extent, caught on: in Korea, Taiwan (where pills are advertised in newspapers and can be obtained by mail order), Malaysia, Iran,

Turkey, Latin America (US aid to those countries for birth control purposes has been angrily denounced as 'psychic imperialism'), Ceylon, and throughout Western Europe. Even in staunch Roman Catholic countries such as Spain and France, the attractions of oral contraception have softened traditional objections to birth control. The arrival of the pill was a significant factor in France's relaxation of the law against contraceptive devices, in 1968. In Spain, the pill enjoys a brisk sale and plans have been announced for the manufacture of over forty million oral contraceptives a year in ten Spanish factories; say, enough for over 160,000 women. Even China has a pill: a progestogen-oestrogen mixture copied from the American original. And in Eastern Europe it is the same: contraceptive pills are well established in Hungary, Czechoslovakia, Rumania and Yugoslavia. Only the USSR has maintained an officially stony attitude to the pill. In 1967, in company with nine other British journalists, I was received by the Soviet Health Minister Dr Boris Petrovski, who is also an eminent surgeon. Asked then about his attitude to the pill, Dr Petrovski said, through an interpreter, 'We do not want our children born with deformed hands and feet.' In the Soviet Union, the IUD is preferred – and the Russian authorities are unfashionably concerned about the falling birth-rate.

Something should be said here about the traditional 'barrier' methods. Indeed, in the present state of impasse, they begin to seem a great deal less despicable than they did in the heyday of the contraceptive pill. They have a lot to recommend them – except their comparatively high failure rates. In this respect, the pill's virtually one hundred per cent effectiveness has set a high standard, and large numbers of couples would be satisfied with nothing less. The IPPF cites a rate of two to three pregnancies per hundred woman-years for the barrier methods, if they are used with anti-sperm jellies, pastes or creams, but admits that this is a generous estimate and warns that if motivation is weak, a higher pregnancy-rate must be expected.

Of the two types, the cap has more disadvantages than the condom. The overall failure rate is higher, and having a cap that fits properly means a visit to a doctor or a clinic. Also, though it is a debatable point, slightly more premeditation is required than with the condom. One way and another, the day of the condom is far from done: it may be just dawning, even though it is one of the most venerable forms of birth control.

In condom technology, the last breakthrough, if that is the word, happened in the nineteenth century when vulcanization of rubber was invented, making it possible to manufacture ultra-thin rubber condoms to replace those made of animal skins or linen. Since then nothing of comparable importance has happened in the condom's history, although from time to time the manufacturers introduce variations in shape. One of the latest, with a more bulbous end to fit over the end of the penis, carries with it an excitingly worded promise from the makers, LR Industries Ltd, of 'new thresholds in sensitivity and comfort'.

LR Industries, a giant firm which evolved out of the London Rubber Company (originally a firm of chemists' sundriesmen), now sits in its world headquarters on London's North Circular Road with an air of understandable confidence. Not only do they control most of the world's supply of condoms – or, as they prefer them to be known, protectives – they have also grown into an unexpectedly diversified business, with interests in surgical clothing, household gloves and party balloons, and also liquor (they own Wine Ways, a chain of over 160 wine, beer, spirit and mineral shops), automatic machines and bikini-style paper panties. Nine out of ten condoms bought in Britain are made by LR Industries – they estimate that sales are running at some 700,000 gross a year – and since 1963 they have owned the comparable American firm of Julius Schmid in New York, who also command the Canadian market. They have agents all over the world and (a point in common with G. D. Searle) they now have their own factory in India, turning out around thirty million condoms annually but with a production capacity five times larger.

Right from the beginning London Rubber's attitude to the pill has been equivocal. One of their first reactions was to sponsor a public relations campaign against oral contraceptives through an organization known under the title of the Genetic Study Unit. The Genetic Study Unit mushroomed into life in 1964 with a cyclostyled bulletin announcing a crusade dedicated to 'protecting the women of the world from mass conversion to faith in oral contraceptives'. When the women of the world showed no willingness to be protected, London Rubber did a volte-face and got into the pill business themselves, with a sequential brand – 'Feminor' tablets – based on norethynodrel and mestranol. But their heart cannot have been in it. A package leaflet for 'Feminor' presented it as a product 'for those who do not wish to use normal methods of contraception', and the leaflet for the standard brand of condom talked about 'the method most of us prefer'. LRI spokesmen explain that they brought out 'Feminor' because they wished to offer a comprehensive range of contraceptives: they also make contraceptive caps and IUDs. 'Feminor', however, was one of the high-oestrogen pills covered by the Scowen Committee's cautionary announcement in December 1969, and at this point, with no sign of regret, London Rubber withdrew 'Feminor' from sale.

Of all people LRI had the most cause for satisfaction at the Scowen Committee's caveat. It only confirmed what they had been thinking, and sometimes saying, all along. At a sales conference in a London hotel in 1969 their International Chairman A. R. Reid described the pill as 'a shadow that has lain on us for the past ten or twelve years'. But, he went on, 'in recent months the position has improved. A whole range of serious contra-indications and side-effects have emerged as you well know. But there is still more to come. A lot more'. So things were looking up. And what was more, he told the assembled delegates, it was now possible for the company to advertise in the national Press. At the time of the Scowen Committee's announcement they used this newly-gained opportunity with telling effect, in a series of Sunday newspaper advertisements for their 'Nu-form' condom stressing its safety and convenience ('Nu-form: a contraceptive so harmless it doesn't need a prescription').

There used to be a myth, on the origin of which it is tempting to speculate, that by secret government decree every nth condom in the production line was deliberately punctured in order to discourage promiscuity and perhaps to make sure the birth-rate did not fall too low. Of course it is untrue. Whatever it is that causes the failure-rate of the condom, it can hardly be deficiencies in the condoms themselves. There is an elaborate testing procedure: each condom is put through an electronic system which detects not only the tiniest hole but any potential weakness, and if anything suspicious is found, the condom is automatically rejected. Also every thirty-two seconds a condom falls out of the ranks and disappears into a testing room, where a group of grey-haired ladies in white coats fill the samples with a measured quantity of water and hang them up for three minutes to see if they burst.

London Rubber executives maintain that the condom is the only logical and convenient form of contraception. Perhaps they are right. The condom is certainly simple, and as more than one investigation has proved, the greater a couple's incentive to avoid pregnancy, the lower the failure-rate. Its biggest disadvantage is that even lubricants and new shapes do not entirely make good the loss of sensation. Even with a thickness of one-fiftieth of a millimetre the rubber gets in the way.

A visit to LR Industries' factory at Chingford brings you face to face with human sexuality in a novel way. The sight of those ranks of condom moulds hurrying urgently along the conveyors, dipping themselves in liquid latex and rising erect, is an experience Swift would have found a lot to say about.

But those phallic moulds are not so much obscene as appealing. Whatever else they suggest as they line up to be clothed in their rubber sheaths, they seem to embody the world's impatient desire for a contraceptive free from all doubts about safety and reliability.

Dr Sheldon J. Segal, Director of the Population Council's Bio-Medical Division, describes himself as 'one of the small band of optimists' in the field of world population control. 'I think there has been evidence,' he told me, 'of changes in patterns of fertility in the less developed countries which are a direct result of a concerted and directed effort to bring family planning programmes to these countries. I think that the effects on birthrates, and population growth rates that can be measured now, would not have been seen if there had not been the introduction of family planning programmes in their health services. As far as whether it has made enough of a difference to, essentially, turn off the fuse of the population explosion.... It takes much longer than a few years, and in this field, where you're attempting to change basic modes of human behaviour, ten years is really a very short time. But in the long pull, the start that has been made now has been very important, and in my judgement will be successful.'

If, as one hopes, Segal is right, then the pill could, indirectly at least, take some of the credit in having given a good deal of extra impetus to the work of foundations like the Population Council. The development of the pill gave some hope that the apparently impossible might be achieved. It is possible that future generations of chemical contraceptive may provide an answer in countries where the pill is now an unsuitable method.

# 8. The Experiment Continues

'NEW YORK – *J. George Harrar, PhD, President of the Rockefeller Foundation, said that worldwide experience with newer contraceptives in mass control campaigns had convinced increasing numbers of field workers and population specialists of the need to "go back to the laboratory" for better contraceptive methods. New and improved methods, he said, can come only from intensive and extensive research in basic reproductive biology*' –

Medical Tribune (New York), 6 February 1969

'Mr St John Stevas *(Chelmsford, C) – Would not the best answer be to develop a contraceptive pill which could be taken by men? (Laughter.)*
Mr Robinson – *This might be a solution. Conceivably, this too might have undesirable effects. (Renewed laughter.)*'

The Times, 1 May 1968

Why not a contraceptive pill for men? The idea may have provoked hearty laughter at Westminster but there is nothing outlandish about it, and it is curious that comparatively little has been done to achieve it. Study of the male reproductive system is well advanced, and a man's reproductive organs are easier to work with than a woman's: the male gonads, the testes, are placed conveniently outside the body, whereas the female gonads, the ovaries, are hidden within. Rough tests of a man's fertility are relatively simple, and the effect of drugs can be readily checked, by taking a sample of his semen.

Yet in only a few laboratories is research going on into ways of controlling male fertility. The British Government has specifically rejected a proposal that funds should be devoted to research on a contraceptive pill for men – influenced perhaps by a Labour Peer who, when the question came up in the House of Lords, urged the government not to take too much notice of 'these do-gooders who take all the fun out of life' (laughter).

One research worker, Dr Harold Jackson of the Christie Hospital, Manchester, has ascribed sluggishness of research into contraception for men to 'particular apprehension regarding the risks involved with tampering chemically with the male germ cells'. Yet tampering chemically with the reproductive system is exactly what is being done in the case of women who take the contraceptive pill, and the risk has been wished on them largely by men. Possibly research on pills for men should be handed over to women pharmacologists. As another researcher – in what is a limited field – Dr Timothy Glover, remarked, 'Our attitude towards sex and research on reproduction is full of tribal beliefs. You come across this if you ask a man to produce a sample of his semen. Now if you ask a rabbit he is only too delighted when you present him with an artificial vagina. But a man will say, "You give me a woman and I'll do it." I say to them, "Well, you've got a hand, haven't you?" But they find this quite distasteful.'

Glover went on:

You would be surprised at the enormous amount of reticence there is in the scientific world about sex and reproduction. There's some antagonism towards sexual physiology as a subject. I was regarded at the outset as someone quite peculiar. There are distinguished physiologists who regard the idea of a male contraceptive as quite repulsive, but they have been working on the female pill all their lives.

Anyway the majority of research workers in reproductive biology have been men. And you know the old story. When students are asked to describe the female reproductive system, the men describe it from the vagina upwards, but the women describe it from the ovaries downwards.

Dr Glover's own research at Liverpool University, with a Ford Foundation grant of £60,000, is on the factors controlling male fertility. Although it might eventually open up new possibilities in male contraception, that is not a specific part of his programme. So far the programme has included a journey to Zambia to study the production and maturation of sperm in what are known as testicond mammals – animals which have their testicles permanently in their abdomens. They interest reproductive biologists because this suggests that they do not require a temperature lower than the rest of the body for the production of viable sperm. Human beings do. The temperature of the scrotum, outside the body, is a few significant degrees lower than inside. Testicond mammals are also intriguing because they have breeding seasons, implying the existence of some mechanism for switching sperm-production on and off according to seasonal need.

Another who regards research into male contraceptives as a neglected area is Dr John Rock, in Boston. He now spends a good part of his time on the problem and has also made use – successfully, he says – of the different temperature requirements of the human testicle to produce a state of temporary infertility. It seems a surprising departure from the course of his best-known work, but he says, 'Not having been a gynaecologist all my life I could handle a man's penis and his balls, and stick my finger up his arse, which no gynaecologist can do.' Rock told me he had one patient whom he had sterilized for periods as long as three months, using a method 'so simple you would laugh – a 150-watt bulb held four to six inches from the scrotum, half an hour a day, for two weeks. What could be simpler?'

Rock went on: 'If that kind of treatment could do it, we went into the use of reinforced jockstraps. We just got a layer of triangles of oilcloth and fitted this into the pouch of one of the modern athletic jockstraps. Wearing that for three weeks would sterilize a man for four to five weeks from the time he started.'

Shortly after this treatment ends, there is a rebound effect when the sperm-count leaps up higher than the average pretreatment figure. When the temperature principle is applied in reverse, and the testicles are not heated but cooled, it has the effect of raising the sperm-count without any intervening period of subfertility. The method is to apply small ice-packs to the scrotum. When Rock and his colleagues used first the heating, then the cooling technique, this produced a double upsurge in sperm-count: therefore, he believes, this could be a suitable treatment for infertility in men.

Unfortunately the results with this method suggest that it may be sub-fertility, not infertility, which is brought about by warming up the testicles for a few minutes each day. Instead of a hundred million sperms per c.c. a man's count might go down to six million, which is a steep fall, but still leaves more than enough sperms to lead to conception if intercourse takes place at the critical time. Something more reliable is required, and from time to time hopeful-sounding reports circulate of new compounds which might produce the foundation for a genuine oral contraceptive for men. But so far none of these has reached the stage of serious clinical trial.

A particular disappointment was one with the cryptic name WIN 18,446. When tested on convict-volunteers it proved effective as a suppressor of sperm-production and, apparently, quite harmless. It was also cheap. But what the researchers had not bargained for was its effects in combination with alcohol. If a man took the drug and then had a drink, his heart raced and he vomited, and some of the men were gripped with unreasonable terror – an effect similar to that of antabuse, a drug used to treat alcoholism. Dr Edward Tyler in Los Angeles described the effects of WIN 18,446 in the following way: 'When one of our first volunteers, a truck driver, stopped for lunch and had a beer and took his pill, it produced the same effect as if he had downed a fifth of Hennessey's Scotch within about two minutes. This created an interesting situation when he carooned off the crowded freeway in his truck, following what we scientifically term a scattergram.' To put paid to the doctors' hopes for this compound, it was also discovered that it damaged the liver.

If the cue were to be taken from the present oral contraceptives prescribed for women, a male pill would attempt to control sexual function at the level of the pituitary, by interfering with hormone balance so that sperm-production, like ovulation in the female, was smothered. Why not a pill which instead of the female hormone oestrogen, contained the male equivalent, androgen? It has been tried, and it does depress fertility, but it depresses libido as well, makes the testicles shrink and the breasts grow. But assuming that this could not be overcome by the type of molecular manipulation that produced the original synthetic steroids, there are other stages in the male reproductive process which could be interrupted: for instance, the development of sperms from their precursors, the spermatids, or the processes involved in their nutrition, or their passage along the minute tubes inside the testes, a stage which takes about two weeks, at the end of which the sperms are mature. Or it might be possible to find a way of interfering at the stage when the sperms are mixed with seminal fluid, from which they derive protection and sustenance. Many of these processes are only partly understood, but if experience with contraceptives for women is any guide, this should not be any deterrent.

Human sperms are remarkable things, and it is understandable that biologists who work with them become highly enthusiastic on the subject. 'I could sit and watch them all day long through the microscope,' said Dr Glover. 'The sperm is a fascinating cell to work with. It leads an independent existence, with its own metabolism. It's mobile, and self-propelling, and that's a fairly unique situation in mammalian cells you know.'

Not only this, but sperms contain the male's share of the normal forty-six chromosomes needed to pass on hereditary characteristics when one of them unites with the ovum. But before the sperm penetrates the ovum it passes through a little-understood stage known as capacitation, again a point at which some contraceptive method might be applied. Freshly ejaculated sperms are not capable of fertilizing an ovum and they can only do so after they have spent some hours in the female tract. But whether capacitation is due to some internal change within the sperm, or to some agent present in the vagina, cervix or uterus, is not clear. But it has proved possible to bring about capacitation by incubating sperms in fluid taken from the female tract, and this might lead to methods of identifying exactly what causes the process. Some progress has also been made in clarifying what happens when a sperm makes its way into the ovum: it appears that some kind of signal reaches the sperm from the ovum and this helps break down the cap-like structure at the sperm's head.

Still another line of inquiry comes from the fact that sperm can be decapacitated, after capacitation has taken place, by incubating them in, surprisingly, seminal fluid – which brought them into the female tract in the first place. The man who showed this was so, in rabbits, bulls and men, was Pincus's co-worker at the Worcester Foundation, Dr Min-Chueh Chang. His discovery has led to a search for a 'decapacitation factor', and if this could be identified, it might lead to the discovery of a natural male contraceptive agent of a most accurate kind. A group of doctors at the University of Georgia are now said to be 'going all out' to track this factor down: and among other things they have managed to induce recapacitation – sperms which have been first made capable of fertilization, then 'defused', and finally had their full potency restored.

One of the dangers involved in meddling with the production, storage, transport or capacitation of sperm is that it might lead to ova being fertilized by sperms that were defective, so-resulting in deformities in the foetus. There are after all immense numbers of sperms to be considered: between two hundred and five hundred million may be carried into the vagina during a single ejaculation.

But the general feeling among research workers is cautiously hopeful, a feeling no doubt enhanced by the understandably keen interest taken by the drug companies. One of these, Upjohn, is known to be experimenting with a chemical which has been nicknamed 'the dynamite pill' because it contains nitroglycerol, a constituent of explosives. But this is only one of a number of chemicals found capable of interfering with various stages of sperm production in mammals, a fact which has led Dr Harold Jackson, for instance, to say that, in the circumstances, 'a prophecy that many other such compounds exist would not seem to be unduly optimistic'.

However, there can only be a slim chance that a marketable drug will emerge within, say, five years from such research as is under way. But now that the female oral contraceptives are less favourably regarded, research on contraceptives for men is getting a much-needed boost. For, as far as contraceptives for women are concerned, matters now seem to have reached dead-lock.

The withdrawal of the progestogen-only drugs, the 'mini-pills' 'Normenon' and 'Verton', was a heavy blow to more people than the manufacturers and the consumers. For research workers also, the 'mini-pill' was the light that failed. When I visited New York in the spring of 1969 the low-dose progestogen 'Normenon', then on the verge of being marketed in Britain, was being spoken of at the Population Council as 'the only real advance in oral contraception'. These pills did not prevent ovulation, but in all probability had some effect on the mucus in the cervix, making it a hostile environment for sperms – slowing them down and even, probably, making the cervical mucus impenetrable. The advantages of the 'mini-pill' in reversing the blood-clotting action of the classical pills, and their apparent lack of effect on blood-sugar level have already been mentioned. Clinical trials of the low-dose progestogen chlormadinone were also at that time showing encouraging results, more so than later on. Although some of the women had had chaotic menstrual cycles, the contraceptive effectiveness of the compound had been shown to be nearly as complete as that of the classical pills. But trials in Britain showed that, for British women at least, this was not so; nevertheless 'Normenon' was sanctioned by the Drug Safety Committee and formally released for prescription in May 1969. Eight months later Syntex in Britain voluntarily withdrew it. E. R. Squibb, makers of 'Verton', followed suit. Syntex's withdrawal of the drug exasperated some research workers, who thought the firm's policy-makers far more agitated than the research results justified: extrapolating the results from beagles to human subjects was unwarranted. Syntex's medical director, Dr George Christie, pleading that in a field of 'partisan medical opinion' they had to err on the side of extreme caution, said, 'We are dealing with a hysterical overaction in the public and in this climate the decision could not have been otherwise.' A few months later, in April 1970, Syntex announced that it did now seem that results in women were different from those in dogs, and that tests on beagles were particularly misleading. In the circumstances, 'Normenon' would be returned to the market as soon as these findings became certain – not later than the end of 1970 (a promise that was not kept).

Temporary or permanent, the demise of the 'mini-pill' meant that the most promising avenue of research now looked a good deal less promising. It would have been difficult to entertain the encouraging thought, voiced by a Population Council official, that if there ever should be a ban on the older oral contraceptives, the low-dose progestogens would be waiting in the wings. The withdrawal of 'Normenon' could set contraceptive research back ten years. It is true that Syntex's own progestogen, chlormadinone (the active ingredient in 'Normenon' and 'Verton'), was only one of several agents under trial, reports on which have now and again surfaced in the medical press. But it is doubtful whether in the present state of opinion drug companies or research foundations will be anxious to spend more money on this particular drug 'family'.

A number of research workers have tried to get over the problems of low-dose continuous treatment (poor control of the menstrual cycle and inadequate contraceptive effect) by using long-acting injectable preparations of progestogen. The injections last three months, and, with a bigger dose, six months. A similar idea has been tried using progestogen and synthetic oestrogen as well, in injections lasting one month, so that this regimen is really the equivalent in a syringe of the present-day oral pill. The resourceful Dr Edward Tyler first started work on injectable preparations as long ago as 1962. At the prescribed intervals, the woman presents herself at the surgery to be injected in the buttocks with a new dose of synthetic hormones and does not have the trouble of remembering to take her daily pill. There have been conflicting reports on how effective the injection method is, though it is at least as good as low-dose progestogen-only pills in this respect. With the three-month or six-month injections, as might have been expected, the effect on the menstrual cycle was even more chaotic than with the 'mini-pill'. Some women who took part in a trial with the four-times-a-year regimen had their periods ten times within twenty-two weeks, others had them ten times within eighteen months. Some women bled for six days, some for twenty. Some women would stop bleeding, only to start again three days later, while others would go as long as 146 days before they bled again. When they stopped having the injections, nearly all the women started to ovulate once more, but not for a while – there was usually a six-month delay before ovulation resumed. Some had to wait longer than a year. Small wonder that, apart from bleeding irregularities, the main complaint voiced by the women was 'nervousness'. There were 216 in this particular trial, and all of them had joined willingly – in preference to using any of a variety of traditional and modern methods of contraception, including monthly injections.

Altogether the injection method does not sound promising. Its cost is another argument against it, and some doctors feel contraception-by-injection would be unacceptable because the whole thing becomes too much trouble. Not all think this way: one population expert remarked that the method at least had the advantage of according with the most popular image of what a doctor ought to be – a man in a white coat holding a full hypodermic.

A slightly different approach is the use of 'Silastic' capsules, implanted under the skin and containing a low-dose progestogen which is absorbed in minute quantities over a period of up to three years. Theoretically it would not interfere with ovulation but have some effect on the sperm's journey through the female tract. The actual implantation procedure is not very complicated because the capsules are very small: they have been compared with threads, cigarette filters and even microscopic dots. If they are small enough these devices could be placed in position, in the buttocks or the arm, by a needle. A similar method has been successfully used in the past as a treatment for diseases needing prolonged dosage.

Yet another idea is a progestogen-impregnated ring, to be put into the vagina and left for twenty-eight days at a time. This quoit-shaped device measures about three inches in diameter, but according to Dr Daniel R. Mishell of Los Angeles County

Harbour General Hospital, who has given it to eighteen women, it does not get in the way during intercourse and neither husbands nor wives have complained. But some of the several varieties of ring have proved uncomfortable to wear all the time, and also there was clear evidence that they suppressed ovulation. Thus the method does not achieve the sought-after local effect, but causes more fundamental changes which are likely to have greater side-effects.

Of all the ideas circulating around research establishments, the most appealing is a 'morning-after' pill, also called the 'just in case' or post-coital pill. The idea is based on the fact that the hormones produced in the ovary are known to play a role in the implantation of the fertilized ovum: therefore by upsetting the hormone environment at the time when the ovum was bedding down in the uterus, one could put a stop to the process. Before he died Pincus was working on steroid compounds which were known to prevent implantation if taken by animals after they had mated. With some animals there is a sudden surge of oestrogen output at this time, and for this reason some of the work on after-intercourse pills has been done with drugs acting against oestrogen. But synthetic oestrogens themselves might be used on the principle that extra quantities would sufficiently alter the local balance of hormones. This has been tried in a small number of cases – some of them women who had been raped – and there have been no pregnancies.

For some people a post-coital pill suggests a do-it-yourself abortion, but the kind of drug on which the reproduction scientists have been working is not quite that: it prevents implantation rather than de-implanting an already secure embryo. One hazard that has been suggested with any drug of this kind is that it might not work completely, and that the embryo could implant itself in the womb in a state which could lead to a deformed foetus. Yet the research people continue to look for a drug which might have the desired effect and no others, despite numerous setbacks and disappointments. In Sydney University's Veterinary Physiology Department they have investigated at least 150 compounds since the early fifties which might form the basis of a morning-after pill. Professor Clifford

Emmens, who heads the department, regards post-coital contraception as one of the next likely advances in fertility control. He also believes such a drug should be taken only at regular, defined periods in the month, when implantation might be expected to occur, rather than every time intercourse had taken place – a routine which might amount to more or less continuous dosage and therefore have some of the disadvantages of the present oral contraceptives.

What could be a major drawback to much of the research, whether on pills for men or women, is that the drugs used are members of the same steroid family that has already led us into difficulties. It has been said that the success of the first generation of oral contraceptives has actually held up progress in research since then, by concentrating people's efforts on what are basically variations of the same theme. 'Oral contraception has reached an impasse,' wrote one expert recently, Dr Arnold Klopper of Aberdeen University, 'where a radically new idea is needed – preferably a technique that does not involve as much endocrine insult as does the present generation of compounds.' But no method which relies on the steroids – 'those thoroughly nasty drugs,' as one British research worker called them – offers a very clear way out. At the Population Council's Bio-Medical Division a determined effort is being made to break away from the steroids in a programme which includes an investigation of 'anti-progestational' drugs. This need not involve the steroids at all. At the end of a menstrual cycle in which there has been no conception, the corpus luteum (the gland which produces progesterone) is, in certain animals but not necessarily in human beings, broken down by a lysin, or a kind of solvent, synthesized in the womb. If conception has taken place, the lysin is not produced. If this solvent could be isolated in human beings and made in the laboratory, it could provide a way of ending a pregnancy almost as soon as it has begun.

There is evidence that this power to destroy the corpus luteum might be possessed by the prostaglandins. Prostaglandins are intriguing substances. What is more, they are the most likely cause of the next pharmaceutical gold rush.

Prostaglandins are found in many body tissues, and (as their name rather tortuously implies) in human semen. Thirteen different prostaglandins had been identified by the end of 1969 but there was a general expectation that more were awaiting discovery. The first were in fact discovered in the 1930s, but it was not until 1968, when a group of Harvard University scientists succeeded in synthesizing five of them that research on prostaglandins became possible on a major scale.

Among their actions on the body as a whole is stimulation of smooth muscle. They also lower blood pressure. This combination of effects has led to the belief that medicine (and the drug industry) may be about to be presented with a whole new and potent family of naturally occurring drugs, capable of treating illnesses as diverse as high blood pressure and heart disease, kidney disease, stomach ulcers, asthma and even nasal congestion.

Nevertheless it is the contraceptive usefulness of prostaglandins which, so far, has been exploited the most. They had already been used to bring on labour at the end of pregnancy when in January 1970, two doctors reported in the *Lancet* that they had terminated fourteen pregnancies by infusing a prostaglandin into the women's veins. The infusions caused contractions of the womb and consequent expulsion of the foetus, though they also caused vomiting and diarrhoea in some of the women, who had been pregnant for periods from nine to twenty-two weeks. Matters advanced so quickly that by the autumn of 1970 tests were taking place in Sweden in which thirty women were using prostaglandins as their sole means of birth control, and in Britain controlled trials of prostaglandins, given by injection, were under way for the Committee on Drug Safety. At a conference on prostaglandins in New York, attended by over 500 scientists from all over the world, Dr Reimert Ravenholt, of the Office of Population in the Agency for International Development, gave voice to the excitement felt by many research workers. 'Something has finally come along,' he said, 'that is very close to a non-toxic, self-administrable, completely effective, once-a-month contraceptive that can be used with the practice of hindsight.' It was almost 'the ultimate means of fertility control'.

Meantime, while the world awaits realization of these hopes, gradual steps forward have been made in understanding the substances that the embryo needs as a source of energy. In rabbits, as well as other species, it is known that at least one specific protein, called blastokinin, is needed for the embryo to grow. If this could be made inactive, it would be a significant step forward, because it is the embryo's own private protein and does not seem to have any other functions. In this case inactivating blastokinin would be unlikely to damage other body systems. It suggests a highly accurate contraceptive method – but at present, only for rabbits. Blastokinin has not yet been identified in man.

It is also possible that the body's reaction to foreign tissue might be put to use in contraception. Could women be made immune to sperm, or to some other natural substance involved in pregnancy? It sounds implausible, but it already happens in certain rare instances. A girl whose case was described in a specialist medical journal in 1967 had an acute allergic reaction to a constituent in human sperm: she came from a family with a long history of various kinds of allergy, including eczema, asthma and dermatitis. After her first sexual experience she developed a generalized rash and asthma; her lips, eyelids, tongue and throat became swollen, she had violent pains in the pelvis and finally lost consciousness. She had most of these symptoms every time she had intercourse: they came on within half an hour and lasted well into the next day. So intense was the girl's reaction that when semen diluted to one part per million was injected under her skin, it left an angry weal.

Some doctors believe reactions of this kind, though a great deal less violent and upsetting, may explain cases of otherwise inexplicable barrenness. Likewise some cases of infertility in men have been attributed to the fact that by a freak of nature they develop antibodies against their own sperms. There are natural precedents, however uncommon, for the effects which physiologists are working for in what is becoming known as 'immunoreproduction'. The Population Council regards this approach to birth control as one of the most promising. A number of possibilities are being studied: immunizing men against their own sperms; and immunizing women against sperms;

immunizing women against the tissues produced in pregnancy such as placenta or umbilical tissue; and immunizing men and women against the gonadotrophins – agents which stimulate the sex-glands – thus inhibiting respectively manufacture of sperm and the development of follicles.

The first two of these approaches have had the most attention so far. Scientists have been able to induce what is technically called allergic aspermatogenesis in whole series of guinea-pigs, by injecting them with material prepared from the testicles of a member of their own species. 'With one immunization,' said Dr Kenneth A. Laurence, Associate Director of the Population Council's Bio-Medical Division, 'we can get ejaculates free of sperm for six months. After that, they recover, and can produce normal offspring, no question about it. And the most encouraging thing is, they never lose their sex drive. The treatment has no influence on androgen production, and they certainly mate if they can.'

The drawback, Laurence explained, was that to achieve this temporary infertility it was necessary to use an adjuvant – a factor added to the injected material to enhance production of antibody. 'If you inject this,' he said, 'you get a severe lesion below the skin, which would never be acceptable to men, and to this day we have never been able to find a practical substitute. It has been tried on men. Mancini in Buenos Aires did it. His patients were men with cancer of the prostate who were due to be castrated, and they volunteered. The effect of the adjuvant was exactly the same in the human as in the guinea-pig.'

There is another problem with the treatment: it produces atrophy of the testes. In guinea-pigs at the time of immunization, the average testicular weight was 2 grammes. Two months later the average weight had gone down to 300 milligrammes. The condition is not permanent, but the psychological effect of having one's testicles reduced to one-seventh their proper size can be imagined. ('I don't think there's a man in the world would appreciate *that*,' Laurence said.)

Some men who are infertile already possess a factor which causes their sperms to clump together so that they are incapable of fertilizing anything. Conceivably one could identify this clumping factor and inject it into men who wished to be made infertile. But when this condition occurs naturally, it cannot be cured. Therefore in the present state of knowledge, having the injection would be the chemical equivalent of a vasectomy – and just as final.

It may be, as some physiologists maintain, that immunological engineering offers the best hope for future methods of birth control, but if so it will not be in the near future. Even farther off than this, however, is control of reproduction by pheromones.

Pheromone is a word coined in 1959 to describe substances used by insects for purposes of sexual attraction. But it has now come to apply to mammals, birds and fish as well. Pheromones are chemicals that are smelled, tasted, or sometimes just absorbed. But most of those that have been identified so far are olfactory pheromones, concerned with smell, with most attention given to the ones which affect sexual behaviour. (There are in addition aggression pheromones, status pheromones, and keep-off-my-land pheromones.) Many pieces of evidence have been collected which fill out the common observation that in the animal world, with the exception of man, life revolves around what you can smell, and only to a limited extent what you see and hear. For instance, if a female cat is put into a cage which has been occupied by a tom-cat, and not washed out afterwards, she starts to behave as though she were on heat. A ram uses his sense of smell to distinguish between ewes which are on heat and those which are not, and if his sense of smell is blocked out, he cannot discriminate and moves around the flock until by trial and error he eventually finds a ewe to receive him. The pattern seems to be that female animals' sex pheromones are for identification, while the male pheromones have an aphrodisiac effect.

From the reproductive physiologist's point of view, one of the most suggestive discoveries (made by a woman research worker at Cambridge, Miss H. M. Bruce) is the influence that male smells can have on early pregnancy in mice. For the first four days after she has mated, that is to say before implantation of the embryo, a female mouse is still vulnerable to the smell of a male. So much so that if a second male comes along, she may be so influenced by his pheromones that the pregnancy fails, the embryo is not implanted and she comes on heat again – and will take the second male for a mate and bear his litter. Female mice which have had their sense of smell inactivated do not succumb to the smell of strange mice after intercourse. But with some female mice whose sense of smell is intact, it does not even need the physical presence of a second male to nip pregnancy in the bud. It can be done by putting the mouse in a cage soiled by male mice, or exposing her to male urine, or even by merely exposing her to air which has passed over male mice.

One can only dimly imagine this curious phenomenon ever being applied to human beings, still less harnessed to some contraceptive purpose. But it is possible that some such process as has been seen in mice was at work in the experiments by Dr Richard Michael, using monkeys, which were described on pages 136–8. An odd footnote to these discoveries can be found in the experience of a Canadian doctor when he perpetrated an innocent joke in a medical journal. It illustrates both the gullibility of some drug manufacturers and their eagerness to find something new in contraception. The doctor, a certain Dr J. S. Greenstein, published a paper on a fictitious contraceptive which he called 'Armpitin', for which he sketched the chemical formula, including several molecular groups represented by the jocularly significant initials NO. 'Armpitin', he explained, was found to affect males by way of the olfactory nerve, and rendered them sterile for a number of days equivalent to the number of NO groups in the formula. Unfortunately the paper was seriously reviewed in an annual review of pharmacology. Dr Greenstein was surprised to receive a number of requests from pharmaceutical companies abroad to sell them the patent.

Unless somebody, one of the drug companies perhaps, has an ace concealed, which seems very unlikely, the immediate future in contraceptive research looks discouraging.

Whatever form new contraceptives take, the major lesson learnt from the first decade of the 'contraceptive revolution' is that the simpler they are, the better. One hope, perhaps, is the C-film, described in *World Medicine* as 'the first his-and-hers contraceptive'. It represents the first practical new idea since the invention of the pill, and consists of a thin, transparent, flexible film about 1½-inches square impregnated with a sperm-killing chemical of which the formula has not yet been published. Men or women can use it. A man has to put it on the end of his penis just before intercourse, so that when he penetrates the vagina the C-film is placed in the position where sperms will be deposited. Women can use it either just before intercourse or up to three hours before: they merely have to push it into the vagina. The film begins dissolving at once and makes the cervical mucus impenetrable to sperms, but the spermicide does not become thin enough to run out, and women can walk about with the film in place.

C-films are cheap. They have been on general sale (no prescription needed) in Hungary since December 1968 and cost the equivalent of 1½p each. *World Medicine*'s Editor Dr Michael O'Donnell reported that more than 100,000 Hungarian couples were using them by November 1969 and that the results of a three-year trial with 720 highly fertile couples gave a pregnancy-rate of 3·4 per hundred woman-years. Some of the failures were believed to have been due to women not using the films properly, but this failure-rate would make this method at least as efficient as 'mini-pills' or condoms. C-films are now on trial in at least ten countries, including Britain, under the auspices of the International Planned Parenthood Federation.

So far, no side-effects have been reported with this method, and it has the needed simplicity of the established methods of birth control.

Whether we can break out of the present impasse is up to the research scientists. Progress in medicine is rapid, and the population problem makes a powerful incentive: and it would be surprising if research on new contraceptives had produced nothing by 1980. Yet there is little immediate prospect of a solution being found. Meanwhile, what happens?

The sagacious Dr Christopher Tietze had some relevant

reflections in an article published towards the end of 1968. When I went to see him, he read them to me, while in a schoolyard outside his open window a shouting, laughing horde of children made an obtrusive and not inappropriate background to our talk. Reviewing the statistics of side-effects with the pill, Tietze had written:

Some of us feel that a contraceptive method must be absolutely harmless. I feel that this is not a reasonable position to take. Nor am I primarily concerned with the relative risks to life or health of oral contraceptives versus the reproductive process itself. The evaluation of these risks may easily degenerate into a sort of numbers game based on highly arbitrary assumptions.

It is my belief that human beings have always been willing to take risks to life and health in order to achieve goals or to obtain benefits they consider important. We ride automobiles and airplanes. We smoke cigarettes. We engage in hazardous forms of sports and athletics. And so on and so forth.

To control the number and spacing of pregnancies by a highly effective and highly convenient method, such as oral contraception, is a goal many persons consider very important and thus they are willing to accept the relatively small hazards to life and health it entails. And who but the individuals concerned can say that the benefit is not worth the risk?

The outlook for the pill has become darker since those words were written. Nevertheless, with all its disadvantages, steroid contraception looks like remaining a fact of twentieth-century life for some time: but a fact which will become increasingly difficult to live with, as women continue to take their chance with the pill, though with a greater feeling of unease. A likely tendency is a drift towards use of the intra-uterine device, more and more sterilization operations, and unless something better turns up, a rueful return to the cap and the condom.

It would be ironical if after years of work on the pill and experimenting with other steroids, we were left with nothing much better, in principle, than the contraceptive Casanova used.

Contraceptive revolution may come to seem all too accurate a phrase. The wheel will indeed have revolved – almost full circle.

# Epilogue

*'Do we have a right not to have public hearings and not to make the information available, on the grounds that all the press may not carry it the way some people think they ought to carry it? Or that it is too complicated for the public to understand? ... Or should these matters be made a matter of public knowledge, counting, as it seems we always have to do, upon the ultimate good judgement of the public to come to a reasonable conclusion? Very frequently, in a free country, people do not come to reasonable conclusions. That is no reason for substituting an arbitrary system.... This is one of the risks, it seems to me, of having a free society in which there are many risks'* –

Senator Gaylord P. Nelson, 1970

Had a demonstration been needed of the intensity of feeling which discussion of the pill can generate, it was amply provided in the early weeks of 1970 by a series of hearings which took place before a subcommittee of the United States Senate.

Few events have upset public confidence in the pill more sharply or dramatized so vividly the question of the pill's safety – simultaneously revealing the confusing disagreements over the significance of the information available on the hazards of oral contraception.

Ostensibly, it was the purpose of the inquiry to discover whether women were being adequately informed about the risks of the pill. The 'court' (the hearings had some of the atmosphere of a public trial) was the Monopolies Subcommittee of the Senate Committee on Small Business, a subcommittee originally intended to investigate monopolistic tendencies and their encroachment upon the livelihood and independence of the small businessman. It seems an incongruous setting, for pill contraception is hardly a field for the smalltime operator. However, the Chairman of the subcommittee, Senator Gaylord

P. Nelson, Democratic Senator from Wisconsin, had since 1967 been conducting an inquiry into monopolism in the drug industry. A special investigation of the pill had been planned for some time, he said later, but had been postponed 'simply because I knew it was a sacred cow'.

A few days beforehand, Senator Nelson issued a lengthy statement in justification of the coming investigation and in which he might be thought to have prejudged its outcome, for he accused the Food and Drug Administration and the pharmaceutical companies of having failed to provide doctors and patients with adequate information on the adverse effects of the pill. The Chairman of the FDA's Advisory Committee on Obstetrics and Gynaecology, said the Senator, had said the pill was safe within the meaning of the law. Commissioner Herbert Ley had described the committee's second report (published in the summer of 1969) as favourable. Yet these comforting words had been uttered despite 'doubts and warnings' voiced elsewhere – Senator Nelson quoted as examples a leading article in the *Lancet* and certain passages in the report of the advisory committee itself. Pamphlets produced by the manufacturers made light of the pill's minor dangers and did not even mention the major causes for concern. The public had been exposed to numerous books, reports and declarations about the risks and the efficacy of the pill. In consequence, 'the public is confused'.

It is debatable whether the final effect of the Nelson investigation was to dissipate this confusion or to deepen it. An immediate result, revealed in a poll conducted by *Newsweek* a few days after the hearings began, was that nearly one-fifth of the estimated total of 8,500,000 American women taking the pill stopped doing so. At least twenty per cent of those who were still taking it confessed that their loyalty was wavering: they were giving 'serious consideration' to discontinuing oral contraceptives, and of the eighteen per cent who had already stopped, one-third gave as their reason the hearings before the Senate subcommittee.

This was not a surprising outcome after a week in which a succession of expert witnesses summarized the medical argument against oral contraception and confronted the pill-taking public, no less than the subcommittee, with evidence of the pill's dangers. That the evidence was differently interpreted by various experts made no difference. Admittedly, the testimony included little that was fresh to any assiduous reader of the medical journals. But much of it would have been disturbingly fresh to the average pill consumer, vaguely aware of a slight risk of blood clotting and, perhaps, that there was talk of a possible link between cancer and the pill. The broad range of side-effects, discussed in earlier chapters of this book, is unfamiliar territory, and it was this which was baldly presented to the newspaper-reading, television-watching public by the Washington hearings of January 1970.

Any doctor or pill manufacturer who prized the consumer's confidence in oral contraceptives must have been thoroughly disquieted by the very opening of the proceedings. Before a crowded hearing room, Dr Hugh J. Davis, of Johns Hopkins University School of Medicine, informed the subcommittee that 'the widespread use of oral contraceptives, such as has developed in the United States in the past ten years, has given rise to health hazards on a scale previously unknown to medicine'. Millions of American women were 'consuming these compounds almost as automatically as chickens eating corn', unaware that they might cause serious illness. The public believed oral contraceptives were no more than innocent, natural female hormones, said Dr Davis, who is Assistant Professor of Obstetrics and Gynaecology at Johns Hopkins, but in fact they were synthetic chemicals twenty to forty times as potent as the natural substances. The widespread use of the pill amounted to 'a massive endocrinologic experiment' with millions of healthy women, for the long-range effects might not make their appearance for fifteen or even twenty years – metabolic effects potentially capable of causing arteriosclerosis as well as 'the nagging spectre of cancer'. In the circumstances, no wonder Dr Davis considered it 'extremely unwise to officially license, sponsor and encourage a long-range experiment such as we now have in progress'. But should the pill be banned? No – these agents, he said, were valuable in gynaecological practice, and in any case they should be available as contraceptives for women who would not or could not use other methods of birth control.

Witness after witness spoke with the same scepticism, or some would say pessimism, as Dr Davis. Professor Victor Wynn sumarized his findings in relation to sugar metabolism and blood fats, informing the subcommittee that they would shortly be able to read an as yet unpublished report showing what some had already suspected, that the pill could cause coronary thrombosis. The head of the Cell Biology Branch of the FDA's Bureau of Science, Dr Marvin Legator, spoke of the possibility of genetic defects in babies born after their mothers had been taking the pill. Dr James Whitelaw, of San José, California, explained the risks of a period of infertility after the pill had been discontinued. Dr Roy Hertz set out the evidence for a link between the pill and cancer ('Oestrogen is to breast cancer,' he told the subcommittee, 'what fertilizer is to a wheat crop'). And evidence was given by Dr Philip A. Corfman, Director of the Center for Population Research at the National Institute of Child Health and Human Development, that preliminary findings from a Government-sponsored inquiry suggested that women who decided to use the pill could be more prone to cancer than those who did not. His evidence was dramatically interrupted by a group of women representing Washington Women's Liberation who, to the televised discomfiture of the chairman, protested at 'unsafe contraceptives foisted on uninformed women for the profit of the drug and medical industries – and for the convenience of men'.

The tension which had by this time been created began to show not only in the hearing room but beyond it, in a slump in sales of the pill. But on the central question which the subcommittee had announced its intention of considering – whether women were told enough of these hazards – there was the predictable polarization of views. Dr Joseph W. Goldzieher maintained that the question whether the pill was safe or not should be decided between the patient and her physician, not in the public press. He opposed the publication of information about the pill's adverse effects in the newspapers: 'The patient is not well served,' he declared, 'by being asked to be his own diagnostician, by being given a list of possible complaints and dangers'. Goldzieher went on:

It is by no means certain that a particular woman should use the pill in preference to some other contraceptive device. If she is the type of person who cannot be counted on to take pills regularly or if she hates to take pills in general, this must be known. Medical contraindications to taking the pill can only be determined by a physician. It is also up to a physician to determine to what extent that particular woman is able to participate effectively in the decision-making process and what amount and type of information she can successfully assimilate.

But from the opposing side, Dr Edmond R. Kassouf of Cranford, New Jersey, stated that in his view full disclosure to the patient of the hazards of oral contraception was 'desirable and morally necessary, as the pill represents a mass experiment'. (However, the disclosure should not become an escape device by which the physician shifted on to the patient the final responsibility of taking the pill.) Many women, he conceded, were ill-equipped by experience and temperament to make a judgement he admitted to be difficult. But still, pamphlets distributed by the drug industry and intended for the patient's consumption often made light of the pill's adverse effects. 'Some of the pamphlets mislead and misinform,' he said. 'Others are frankly dangerous. But all have one thing in common. They all seem to disparage their reader's right to know.'

The patient's right to know is what the Nelson hearings were basically all about, but the questions they raised cannot be easily answered. And this public debate focused attention on an issue by no means peculiar to oral contraception but especially relevant to it. Has the patient a right to know? The traditional answer would be: only as much as is good for him. But the more information patients pick up about illness and its treatment, however incomplete or inaccurate it may be, the more difficult it is to satisfy them with vague, if well-intentioned, reassurances. In the case of the pill it is frequently the advocates of oral contraception who are against a full explanation of the side-effects and possible risks of the medication. The sceptics are more often those who believe it necessary to come clean. The ideal state of affairs is suggested by Senator Nelson's own view, that the public has 'a right to informed consent' in the question of medical treatment. An intelligent participation in treatment, whether it is drug therapy, surgery or any other measure, is a wholly desirable solution. But just how difficult it is with the pill, a drug on whose effects the prescribers themselves cannot agree, the Nelson hearings again and again demonstrated.

Doctors who argue, for instance, that too much information can be evil had their views confirmed later in the hearings when it came the turn of Dr Elizabeth Connell to give evidence. The publicity generated by the investigation, she told the subcommittee, had caused panic among women using the pill, leading to dozens of unwanted pregnancies. Speaking to the subcommittee at the end of February, she declared: 'We are just beginning to see the first of the pregnancies of women who panicked in January, stopped using their pills and did not seek or use another means of birth control.' The next day Dr Alan F. Guttmacher, head of Planned Parenthood, who had protested at the undue weight given to evidence against the pill, dourly predicted a sharp rise in the number of abortions, including abortion deaths, and a bulge in the 1971 birth-rate as a result of the Nelson hearings. He was not accusing the subcommittee of any diabolic purpose, he said, 'but there is a tremendous amount of undigested pabulum that comes out in the daily press'. But should women be given more information about the pill's side-effects, Senator Nelson wanted to know? Dr Guttmacher replied: 'The dispenser of therapy should be educated, not the recipient.'

At the subcommittee's session on 4 March it seemed that both recipient and, in a roundabout way, dispenser were indeed to be educated. Dr Charles C. Edwards, the new Commissioner for Food and Drugs, told the subcommittee that steps were to be taken to place in the hands of users of the pill detailed but readily understandable information on the hazards. Yet again, the pill was to be uniquely treated: no other prescription drug carried such explicit warnings as were now proposed for the pill. Commissioner Edwards had come to the conclusion that the information being supplied to the patient was insufficient. And not only did the proposed leaflet, then available in draft form, explain the possible risks of oral contraception, it also made the clear assumption that any woman about to start swallowing her daily pill had been thoroughly examined by her doctor and carefully briefed about its advantages and disadvantages.

'All of the oral contraceptive pills are highly effective for preventing pregnancy', the draft ran, 'when taken according to the approved directions.' It went on:

Your doctor has taken your medical history and has given you a careful physical examination. He has discussed with you the risks of oral contraceptives and has decided that you can take this drug safely.

This leaflet is your reminder of what your doctor has told you. Keep it handy and talk to him if you think you are experiencing any of the hazards you find described.

The draft leaflet continued with a number of specific warnings: that there was a danger of blood clotting, that women who had suffered from serious liver disease, cancer or vaginal bleeding should not take the pill; there were references to the need for special supervision for women who had had heart or kidney disease, asthma, high blood pressure, diabetes, epilepsy, fibroids of the uterus, migraine or mental depression – all of which, it was explicitly assumed, the doctor would already have drawn to the woman's notice. 'Even if you don't have special problems', the leaflet pointedly said, 'he will want to see you regularly to check your blood pressure, examine your breasts and make certain other tests.'

And so it went on, with references to a possible period of infertility if the women stopped using the pill, to the possibility of the pill's ingredients contaminating a nursing mother's milk, to the 'run-of-the-mill' side-effects as well as to mental depression, swelling, skin rash, jaundice, changes in appetite and sex-drive, growth of body hair and loss of hair on the scalp. There was even to be a note about cancer: 'Scientists know the hormones in the pill (oestrogen and progesterone) have caused cancer in animals, but they have no proof that the pill causes cancer in humans. Because your doctor knows this, he will want to examine you regularly.'

The leaflet ended: 'REMEMBER. While you are taking — call your doctor promptly if you notice any unusual change in your health. Have regular check-ups and your doctor's approval for a new prescription.'

At this apparent vindication of his efforts, Senator Nelson was delighted. It was 'a historic and dramatic step' of a kind never taken before, and at the subcommittee hearing on 4 March he told Commissioner Edwards, 'I do commend you for your courage and far-sightedness in doing it. I think this is a great step forward.'

But the Senator spoke too soon. Neither the American Medical Association nor the drug industry shared his satisfaction at the proposed leaflet: the AMA protested that it would interfere with doctor–patient relationships and expose the doctor to the possibility of malpractice suits, while the industry complained that it overemphasized the dangers of the pill and minimized its benefits. The FDA went into reverse. Less than three weeks after publication of the draft, it became known that the leaflet was being toned down. 'The more we got to thinking about it, the more we thought that we had put too much clinical material in it,' Commissioner Edwards explained. 'We decided it wasn't our role to play doctor or to scare people away from the pill.' The detailed catalogue of possible hazards was to be edited out, and the new version soft-pedalled the assumption that the woman reading it had been, or remained, under the vigilant supervision of her physician. The 600 words of the original were being replaced by 100 or so of a more soothing character: 'The oral contraceptives are powerful, effective drugs. Do not take these drugs without your doctor's continued supervision. As with all effective drugs, they may cause side-effects in some cases and should not be taken at all by some.' The original leaflet had said: 'There is a definite association between blood clotting disorders and the use of oral contraceptives. The risk of this complication is six times higher for users than for non-users.' Now the revised version was to read: 'Rare instances of blood clotting are the most important known complications of the oral contraceptives. These points were discussed with you when you chose this method of contraception.'

A little later the FDA announced that it would be obligatory for drug manufacturers to supply doctors with full and detailed information on the known and suspected hazards of oral contraceptives. 'We've put the responsibility back on the physician,' said Commissioner Edwards.

Nevertheless, it seemed the fortunes of the pill had once again fallen only to rise again. A Gallup poll at the end of February had found that after the first sessions of the Nelson hearings roughly two out of three American women believed the pill to be injurious to health – almost an exact reversal of the opinion recorded in a survey three years earlier. (In both surveys, sixty-seven per cent of women said they thought the pill was an effective form of contraception.) But these figures were collected when the unfavourable publicity provoked by the hearings was at the point of maximum impact, and before the counter-balancing effect of the FDA's *volte-face* began to exert any influence. From that moment, one would think, the pill began to recover. It was helped still more by the news from Britain in April: the Drug Safety Committee had finished analysing the evidence which had caused it to recommend British doctors to prescribe only the pills with a low oestrogen content – less than 50 microgrammes. Their deliberations now led them to say that if there were a complete changeover to low-oestrogen pills, the number of deaths from clotting disease among pill-users would be halved, and there would be at least a twenty-five per cent drop in the number of cases of serious but non-fatal clotting disease. Mr Richard Crossman, Secretary of State for Social Services, said at a press conference, 'If your doctor advises you to take the pill, don't be afraid. Take it, because the risk really is minuscule.'

Yet once again the Drug Safety Committee's investigations could have been led astray by incomplete evidence. The 920 reports of thrombosis which formed the basis of their arithmetic were still only a fraction – about ten per cent, it was believed – of the total number of cases that occurred during the period the Committee was interested in. There were some further oddities to be taken into account. It had been found that two brands of pill ('Conovid-E' and 'Previson'), although they contained 100 microgrammes of oestrogen, nevertheless had an unexpectedly low risk of clotting. Why these and not other brands with the same amount of oestrogen? The committee found it hard to explain. Another brand, 'Volidan', contained only the approved 50 microgrammes of oestrogen, but it apparently carried an unexpectedly high risk of blood clotting. Again the reasons for this were mysterious. It could have had something to do with the progestational drugs used in these three brands of pill, or with the way the pills were absorbed in the body, or even with some undetected bias in the figures.

There was another curious finding. It was predictable that there would be a link between the high-oestrogen pills and clotting in the lungs and legs. What was not predictable was that there should also now appear a connection between high-oestrogen pills and coronary thrombosis, the kind of circulatory disease that leads to a heart attack. No conclusive evidence had ever been uncovered in any of the controlled investigations that the pill could cause coronary thrombosis. Could it have been chance that a link had now turned up? Probably not, the authors of the report considered. Could these have been cases of wrong diagnosis – were the women with 'coronary thrombosis' really suffering from clots in the lungs? Again it was unlikely because seventy per cent of the diagnoses had been confirmed by electrocardiography and most of the rest had been reported by hospital doctors. Could it be that there was a real association between coronary thrombosis and the pill which had been consistently missed in the earlier studies? The only answer the authors could give was that further investigation was needed.

Nevertheless the FDA swiftly followed the Scowen Committee's example in Britain, and announced on 24 April that it would be advising physicians to prescribe oral contraceptives low in oestrogen unless the medical needs of the patient dictated otherwise. All the same, FDA officials seemed disposed to be more critical of the Scowen Committee's conclusions than had, for instance, Mr Crossman. One official, Dr John Jennings,

Director of the Bureau of Medicine, was reported as saying that the committee's data had 'severe limitations' and that the three times greater risk of blood clotting with the high-oestrogen pills was 'not terribly impressive'. Further, he believed the 50-microgrammes figure should be treated with caution because of differences in potency among the types of oestrogen used in oral contraceptives on sale in the USA.

About half the total of 8,500,000 American women on the pill were at that time believed to be taking pills with more than 50 microgrammes of oestrogen in them. It seemed more than likely that a swift transition to the weaker-oestrogen pills would, for the time being at least, restore confidence in oral contraception, despite the furore in Washington in the early months of the year. In any case, even without this reassuring development, the pill's advantages would probably have triumphed over the unfavourable publicity generated by the hearings. Even at the height of the scare, an inquiry by the *Wall Street Journal* found evidence that 'many women who genuinely worry about side-effects of the pill are determined to continue using it nevertheless'.

In Britain, it took a mere six months for the figures for pill consumption to climb back to the level of December 1969 (when the Committee on Safety of Drugs issued its warning about pills with a high oestrogen content). The Oral Contraception Information Centre predicted that usage of the pill would continue to increase as before.

An American newspaper reported the comment of a doctor in Dallas, on the pill's worst winter. 'Most of my patients are younger women who just tune out on the criticism. They handle the emotional conflicts the best way they can.'

It is almost the classic reaction. Some would say it is, in the circumstances, the only sensible solution to the personal problem of whether to take the pill or not. A cynic might, on the other hand, compare this reaction to the self-justification of the cigarette smoker. He tunes out on the criticism too. Whether this constitutes a kind of 'informed consent' is another question.

# Index